NURSING THEORIES AND MODELS

Ruby L. Wesley, RN, PhD

Dr. Wesley, author of this book, is a Lecturer at Wayne State University, Detroit. She received her BSN and MEd from Wayne State University and her PhD in nursing from the University of Maryland. Dr. Wesley is a member of Sigma Theta Tau, Lambda Chapter, the American Nurses' Association, the District of Columbia Nurses' Association, and the Midwest Nursing Research Society.

Marylou K. McHugh, RN, EdD

Dr. McHugh, reviewer of this book, is an Assistant Professor of Nursing and Graduate Director, LaSalle University, Philadelphia. She received her diploma in nursing from Pennsylvania Hospital School of Nursing, Philadelphia; her BSN from Gwynedd Mercy College, Gwynedd, Pa.; her MSN from the University of Pennsylvania, Philadelphia, and her EdD from Teachers College, Columbia University, New York. Dr. McHugh is a member of the American Nurses' Association, the Pennsylvania Nurses' Association, the National League for Nursing, the Museum of Nursing History, and Sigma Theta Tau.

Springhouse Corporation
Springhouse, Pennsylvania

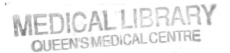
Staff

Executive Director, Editorial
Stanley Loeb

Director of Trade and Textbooks
Minnie B. Rose, RN, BSN, MEd

Art Director
John Hubbard

Clinical Consultant
Maryann Foley, RN, BSN

Editors
David Moreau, Karen Zimmermann

Copy Editor
Mary Hohenhaus Hardy

Designers
Stephanie Peters (associate art director),
Jacalyn Facciolo

Art Production
Robert Perry (manager), Anna Brindisi, Donald
Knauss, Tom Robbins, Robert Wieder

Typography
David Kosten (director), Diane Paluba (manager),
Elizabeth Bergman, Joyce Rossi Biletz, Phyllis
Marron, Robin Rantz, Valerie Rosenberger

Manufacturing
Deborah Meiris (manager), T.A. Landis, Jennifer
Suter

Library of Congress Cataloging-in-Publication Data

Wesley, Ruby L.
  Nursing theories and models / Ruby L. Wesley,
author, Marylou K. McHugh, reviewer.
  p. cm. — (Springhouse notes)
  Includes bibliographical references and index.
  1. Nursing—Philosophy—Outlines, syllabi, etc.
2. Nursing Outlines, syllabi, etc. I. McHugh,
Marylou K. II. Title. III. Series.
  [DNLM: 1. Models, Nursing—outlines.
2. Nursing Theory—outlines.   WY 18 W514n]
RT84.5.W47   1992
610.73'01—dc20
DNLM/DLC   91-4842
ISBN 0-87434-367-4   CIP

Contents

Consultants

Janie Brown, RN, EdD
Dr. Brown is an Associate Professor of Nursing, Villanova (Pa.) University. She received her BS from State University College of New York at Plattsburgh and her MEd and EdD from Teachers College, Columbia University, New York. Dr. Brown is a member of the American Nurses' Association, the Pennsylvania Nurses' Association, the American Association for the History of Nursing, the National League for Nursing, the Museum of Nursing History, the Society for Nursing History, Sigma Theta Tau, Phi Kappa Phi, and Kappa Delta Phi, Kappa Chapter.

Jean Jenny, RN, MEd, MSN
Ms. Jenny is an Associate Professor at the University of Ottawa, Faculty of Health Sciences, Nursing School, Ontario, Canada. She received her BScNEd and MEd from the University of Ottawa and her MSN from the University of California, San Francisco. Ms. Jenny is a member of the Canadian Nurses' Association, Registered Nurses' Association of Ontario, Ontario College of Nurses, North American Nursing Diagnosis Association, and the Provincial Nurse Educators' Association.

How to Use Springhouse Notes

Today, more than ever, nursing students face enormous time pressure. Nursing education has become more sophisticated, increasing the difficulties students have with studying efficiently and keeping pace. The need for a comprehensive, well-designed series of study aids is great, which is why we've produced Springhouse Notes...to meet that need.

Springhouse Notes provide essential course material in outline form, enabling the nursing student to study more effectively, improve understanding, achieve higher test scores, and get better grades.

Key features appear throughout each book, making the information more accessible and easier to remember.
- **Learning Objectives.** These objectives precede each section in the book to help the student evaluate knowledge before and after study.
- **Key Points.** Highlighted in gray throughout the book, these points provide a way to quickly review critical information. Key points may include:
—a cardinal sign or symptom of a disorder
—the most current or popular theory about a topic
—a distinguishing characteristic of a disorder
—the most important step of a process
—a critical assessment component
—a crucial nursing intervention
—the most widely used or successful therapy or treatment.
- **Points to Remember.** This information, found at the end of each section, summarizes the section in capsule form.
- **Glossary.** Difficult, frequently used, or sometimes misunderstood terms are defined for the student at the end of each section.

Remember: Springhouse Notes are learning tools designed to *help* you. They are not intended for use as a primary information source. They should never substitute for class attendance, text reading, or classroom note-taking.

This book, *Nursing Theories and Models,* begins with a historical overview of nursing theory and model development and then chronologically explores 17 renowned nursing theories and models. The text reviews major concepts and assumptions, provides background information on the theorists' education and influences, and analyzes how the theorists address the four concepts of the nursing metaparadigm.

Overview of Nursing Theories and Models

Learning Objectives

After studying this section, the reader should be able to:

- List the information provided by nursing models and theories.

- Define and explain each concept of the nursing meta-paradigm.

- Identify four characteristics of a conceptual model.

- Identify ten characteristics of a theory.

- Trace the historical development of nursing theories and models.

I. Overview of Nursing Theories and Models

A. Introduction
1. The foundation of any profession is the development of a specialized body of knowledge
   a. In the past, the nursing profession relied on theories from other disciplines, such as medicine, psychology, and sociology, as a basis for practice
   b. For nursing to define its activities and develop its research, it must have its own body of knowledge
   c. This knowledge can be expressed as conceptual models and theories
2. Nursing theories and models provide information about:
   a. Definitions of nursing and nursing practice
   b. Principles that form the basis for practice
   c. Goals and functions of nursing
3. Nursing theories and models are derived from concepts
4. A *concept* is an idea of an object, property, or event and can be *empirical* or *concrete* (readily observable, such as a thermometer, bed, lesion, rash, or edema), *inferential* (indirectly observable, such as temperature or pain), or *abstract* (nonobservable, such as health or stress)
5. Conceptual models and theories in nursing are based on the nursing metaparadigm
6. A *metaparadigm* is the organizing conceptual or philosophical framework of a discipline or profession
   a. It defines and describes relationships among major ideas and values
   b. It guides the organization of theories and models for a profession
7. The nursing metaparadigm comprises four concepts: person, environment, health, and nursing
   a. *Person* refers to the recipient of nursing care, including physical, spiritual, psychological, and sociocultural components
   b. *Environment* refers to all the internal and external conditions, circumstances, and influences affecting the person
   c. *Health* refers to the degree of wellness or illness experienced by the person
   d. *Nursing* refers to the actions, characteristics, and attributes of the individual providing the nursing care
8. Theories and models can be categorized according to how they describe, explain, and connect the four concepts of the nursing metaparadigm
9. *Developmental theories and models* emphasize growth, development, and maturation
   a. The primary focus is change in a particular direction
   b. This change is orderly and predictable, occurring in specific stages, levels, or phases
   c. The goal is to maximize growth

10. *Systems theories and models* view persons as open systems
    a. Each open system can receive input from the environment, process it, provide output to the environment, and receive feedback
    b. Each system strives for a *steady state* (balance between internal and external forces)
    c. Change is of secondary importance
11. *Interaction theories and models* are based on the relationships among persons
    a. The primary focus is on the person as an active participant
    b. Emphasis is on the person's perceptions, self-concept, and ability to communicate and perform roles
    c. The goal is achievement through reciprocal interaction
12. The development of nursing theories and models is a relatively recent occurrence
    a. The nursing profession has not reached a consensus on the meaning and interpretation of concepts, theories, and models
    b. A lack of consensus also exists whether a single model or theory should be selected or whether multiple models and theories are more useful to nursing practice
    c. Areas of agreement among theorists include the importance of the four concepts of person, environment, health, and nursing; the goal of enhancing client comfort; a holistic approach of nursing; and a set of distinct values of nursing
    d. Like any profession, nursing must have a theoretical base

B. Models
1. General information
   a. Describe a set of ideas that are connected to illustrate a larger, more general concept
   b. Are a symbolic depiction of reality
   c. Provide a schematic representation of some relationships among phenomena
   d. Use symbols or diagrams to represent an idea
2. Characteristics
   a. Attempt to describe, explain, and sometimes predict the relationships among phenomena
   b. Are composed of empirical, inferential, and abstract concepts
   c. Provide an organized framework for nursing assessment, planning, intervention, and evaluation
   d. Facilitate communication among nurses and encourage a unified approach to practice, teaching, and research

C. Theories
1. General information
   a. Are a set of interrelated concepts that provide a systematic explanatory and predictive view of phenomena

    b. Can begin as an untested premise (hypothesis) that becomes a theory when tested and supported or can progress in a more inductive manner

    c. Are tested and validated through research and provide direction for this research

2. Characteristics

    a. Must be logical, relatively simple, and generalizable

    b. Are composed of concepts and propositions

    c. Interrelate concepts to create a specific way of looking at a particular phenomenon

    d. Provide the bases for testable hypotheses

    e. Must be consistent with other validated theories, laws, and principles but leave open unanswered questions for investigation

    f. Can consist of separate theories about the same phenomenon that interrelate the same concepts but describe and explain them differently

    g. Can describe a particular phenomenon (*descriptive* or *factor-isolating theories*); explain relationships among phenomena (*explanatory* or *factor-relating theories*); predict the effects of one phenomenon on another (*predictive* or *situation-relating theories*); or be used to produce or control a desired phenomenon (*prescriptive* or *situation-producing theories*)

    h. Contribute to and assist in increasing the general body of knowledge within a profession through research implemented to validate them

    i. Can be used by nurses to guide and improve their practice

    j. Differ from conceptual models; both can describe, explain, or predict a phenomenon, but only theories provide specific direction to guide practice; conceptual models are more abstract and less fully developed

3. Levels of theory development

    a. *Meta-theories* focus on broad issues, including analysis of the purpose and type of theory needed, proposal and critique of sources and methods for theory development, and proposal of criteria for theory evaluation (for example, J. Dickoff's and P. James's Theory of Theories)

    b. *Grand theories* (also known as *metaparadigms* or *models*) are abstract in content and broad in scope; they attempt to explain a global view useful in understanding key concepts and principles (for example, D. Orem's General Theory of Nursing or C. Roy's Adaptation Model)

    c. *Middle-range theories* target specific phenomena or concepts, such as pain and stress; they are limited in scope yet general enough to encourage research

    d. *Practice theories* are narrowly defined; they address a desired goal and the specific actions needed to achieve it

D. Historical perspective

1. 1860 to 1959

    a. In 1860, Florence Nightingale developed her Environmental Theory

    b. In 1952, the journal *Nursing Research* was established, encouraging nurses to become involved in scientific inquiry

    c. In the same year, Hildegard Peplau published *Interpersonal Relations in Nursing;* her ideas have influenced later nursing theorists

    d. In 1955, Virginia Henderson published *Definition of Nursing*

    e. In the mid-1950s, Teachers College, Columbia University, New York City, began offering master's and doctoral programs in nursing education and administration, resulting in student participation in theory development and testing

2. 1960 to 1969

    a. During the 1960s, Yale University School of Nursing, New Haven, Conn., defined nursing as a process, interaction, and relationship

    b. Also during the 1960s, the U.S. government began funding master's and doctoral education in nursing

    c. In 1960, Faye Abdellah published *Twenty-One Nursing Problems*

    d. In 1961, Ida Orlando published her theory in *The Dynamic Nurse-Patient Relationship: Function, Process, and Principles of Professional Nursing*

    e. In 1962, Lydia Hall published *Core, Care, and Cure Model*

    f. In 1964, Ernestine Wiedenbach published her theory in *Clinical Nursing: A Helping Art*

    g. In 1965, the American Nurses' Association published a position paper stating that theory development was an important goal for nursing

    h. In 1966, Myra Levine published *Four Conservation Principles*

    i. In 1969, Dorothy Johnson published *Behavioral Systems Model*

3. 1970 to 1979

    a. During the 1970s, Case Western Reserve University, Cleveland, sponsored symposia to stimulate theory development

    b. During the mid-1970s, the National League for Nursing established an accreditation requirement that nursing schools base their curricula on a nursing conceptual framework

    c. In 1970, Martha Rogers published her model in *An Introduction to the Theoretical Basis of Nursing*

    d. In 1971, Dorothea Orem published *Self-Care Deficit Theory of Nursing,* Imogene King published *Theory of Goal Attainment,* and Joyce Travelbee published *Interpersonal Aspects of Nursing*

    e. In 1972, Betty Neuman published *Health Care Systems Model*

    f. In 1976, Sister Callista Roy published *Adaptation Model*

    g. In 1976, J.G. Paterson and L.T. Zderad published *Humanistic Nursing*

    h. In 1978, Madeleine Leininger published *Cultural Care Theory*

    i. In 1979, Jean Watson published *Nursing: Human Science and Human Care—A Theory of Nursing*

4. 1980 to the present

    a. In 1980, Evelyn Adam published *To Be A Nurse* and Joan Riehl-Sisca published *Symbolic Interactionism*

    b. In 1982, Joyce Fitzpatrick published *Life Perspective Model*

    c. In 1983, Kathryn Barnard published *Parent-Child Interaction Model* and Helen Erickson, Evelyn Tomlin, and Mary Ann Swain published *Modeling and Role Modeling*

    d. In 1984, Patricia Benner published *From Novice to Expert: Excellence and Power in Clinical Nursing Practice*

    e. In 1985, Ramona Mercer published *Maternal Role Attainment*

    f. In 1986, Margaret Newman published *Model of Health*

5. Predictions for theory development

    a. The number of theories and models will increase, especially in the middle-range level

    b. The use of nursing theory will be challenged as a result of the nursing shortage and the decreased emphasis placed on nursing theory by the National League for Nursing

    c. Nursing diagnosis will become the leading stimulus for practice theory development

Points to Remember

Theories and models attempt to define and describe the discipline of nursing.

Nursing theories and models provide information about the definition of nursing and nursing practice, principles that form the basis for practice, and the goals and functions of nursing.

The nursing metaparadigm consists of four concepts—person, environment, health, and nursing.

Both theories and models can describe, explain, or predict relationships among phenomena.

Nursing practice must be theoretically based.

The four levels of theory development are meta-theory, grand theory, middle-range theory, and practice theory.

Florence Nightingale was the first nursing theorist.

Glossary

Concept—description of objects, properties, or events that forms the basic components of theory

Metaparadigm—organizing conceptual or philosophical framework of a discipline or profession

Model—symbolic representation of reality, linking groups of concepts and organizing them to formulate a description of a phenomenon

Phenomenon—event, situation, or area of inquiry

Research—systematic, controlled, empirical, and critical investigation of hypothetical propositions about the relationships among natural phenomena

Theory—set of interrelated constructs (concepts, definitions, and propositions) that present a systematic view of phenomena by specifying relationships among variables, with the purpose of explaining and predicting the phenomena

Nightingale's Environmental Theory

Learning Objectives

After studying this section, the reader should be able to:

- List Nightingale's five components of a healthful environment.

- Identify the three types of environment discussed by Nightingale.

- Discuss how Nightingale addresses the four concepts of the nursing metaparadigm.

II. Nightingale's Environmental Theory

A. Introduction

1. Florence Nightingale began her nursing training in 1851 in Kaiserwerth, Germany
2. She pioneered the concept of formal education for nurses
3. Her experience in treating sick and injured soldiers during the Crimean War strongly influenced her philosophy of nursing
4. In 1859, Nightingale published her views on nursing care in *Notes on Nursing;* her ideas continue to form the basis of current nursing practice
5. She is considered the first nursing theorist, although her writings differ in form, tone, terminology, and style from those of contemporary theorists
6. Information on her theory has been obtained through interpretation of her writings
7. Nightingale based her ideas on individual, societal, and professional values
   a. Her strongest influences were education, observation, and hands-on experience
   b. She formulated her ideas and values through years of working with charities and in hospitals and military infirmaries
8. Nightingale's theory has significantly influenced three other theories: Adaptation Theory, Need Theory, and Stress Theory

B. Environmental Theory

1. General information
   a. The foundation of Nightingale's theory is the environment — all the external conditions and forces that influence the life and development of an organism
   b. The interrelationship of a healthful environment with nursing provides the basis for her theory
   c. In Nightingale's era, unsanitary conditions and disease posed a great hazard
   d. According to Nightingale, external influences and conditions can prevent, suppress, or contribute to disease or death
   e. Her goal was to help the patient retain his own vitality by meeting his basic needs through control of the environment
   f. Nightingale described five major components of a positive, or healthful, environment: proper ventilation, adequate light, sufficient warmth, control of effluvia, and control of noise
   g. Although she considered these components necessary for a healthful home, Nightingale was probably also referring to hospitals, workplaces, and the general community (few hospitals existed at that time; most care took place in the homes of the wealthy or in almshouses for the poor)
   h. Nightingale discussed three types of environment: physical, psychological, and social
   i. A patient's physical environment is addressed by keeping records and statistics on mortality and illness in the wards

      j. A patient's psychological and social environments are addressed by providing positive, stress-free surroundings
  2. Physical environment
      a. Consists of physical elements where the patient is being treated, such as ventilation, warmth, cleanliness, light, noise, and drainage
      b. Affects all other aspects of the environment; for example, cleanliness of the physical environment directly relates to disease prevention and patient mortality
      c. Influences a person's psychological environment
  3. Psychological environment
      a. Can be affected by a negative physical environment, which causes stress
      b. Requires various activities to keep the mind active; for example, manual work, appealing food, and a pleasing physical environment help a person survive psychologically
      c. Involves communication with the person, about the person, and about other people; communication should be therapeutic, soothing, and unhurried
  4. Social environment
      a. Involves collecting data about illness and disease prevention
      b. Includes such components of the physical environment as clean air, water, and proper drainage
      c. Consists of a person's home or hospital room, as well as the total community that affects the patient's specific environment

C. Nightingale's theory and the four concepts of the nursing metaparadigm
  1. Person
      a. Referred to by Nightingale as the "patient" in most of her writings
      b. Is a human being acted upon by a nurse or affected by the environment
      c. Has reparative powers to deal with disease; recovery is within the patient's power as long as a safe environment for recuperation exists
  2. Environment
      a. Serves as the foundation of Nightingale's theory
      b. Comprises the external conditions and forces that affect one's life and development
      c. Includes everything from a person's food to a nurse's verbal and nonverbal interactions with the person
  3. Health
      a. Is described by Nightingale as maintaining well-being by using a person's powers to the fullest extent; disease is viewed as a reparative process instituted by nature
      b. Is maintained by controlling environmental factors to prevent disease; health and disease are the focus of the nurse, who helps a person through the healing process

4. Nursing
   a. Aims to provide fresh air, light, warmth, cleanliness, quiet, and a proper diet
   b. Facilitates a person's reparative processes by ensuring the best possible environment
   c. Influences the environment to affect health
   d. Is a discipline distinct from medicine, focusing on the person experiencing a reparative process rather than on the disease of an anatomical structure or the person's physiology
   e. Supports the nursing process (although the latter was formulated many decades after Nightingale's writings)

Points to Remember

Most of the information for Nightingale's theory has been inferred from her writings.

The foundation of Nightingale's theory is the environment.

Nightingale classified the environment as physical, psychological, and social.

She identified five major components of a healthful environment—ventilation, light, warmth, control of effluvia, and control of noise.

According to Nightingale, the function of nursing is to influence the person's environment in ways that will help restore health.

Although Nightingale does not specifically describe the nursing process, her theory supports it.

Glossary

Basic needs—elements required by a person for survival, such as air, water, and food

Effluvia—offensive smells and gaseous odors that must be controlled

Stress—threat or change in the environment to which an individual must adapt

Peplau's Interpersonal Relations Model

Learning Objectives

After studying this section, the reader should be able to:

- Describe Peplau's Interpersonal Relations Model.

- Identify the model's four phases.

- List the roles of the nurse during each phase.

- Discuss how Peplau addresses the four concepts of the nursing metaparadigm.

III. Peplau's Interpersonal Relations Model

A. Introduction

1. Hildegard Peplau began her nursing career in 1931 after receiving a diploma in nursing from Pottstown (Pa.) Hospital School of Nursing
2. In 1943, she received a BA in interpersonal psychology from Bennington College, Vermont
3. In 1947, she was awarded an MA in psychiatric nursing; in 1953, a doctorate in nursing education from Teachers College, Columbia University, New York City
4. She has held positions in the U.S. Army, private and general hospitals, nursing research, teaching, and private practice psychiatric nursing
5. Peplau first published her model in 1952 in *Interpersonal Relations in Nursing*
   a. She referred to this book as a partial theory for nursing practice
   b. The book was reissued in 1988
6. In developing her model, Peplau was committed to incorporating established knowledge into her work
   a. She borrowed from the behavioral sciences and drew from the works of Sigmund Freud, Erich Fromm, Abraham Maslow, Harry Sullivan, and Neal Miller
   b. She integrated psychoanalytical, social learning, human motivational, and personality development theories into her model at a time when nursing theory development was relatively new

B. Interpersonal Relations Model

1. General information
   a. Peplau bases her model on psychodynamic nursing, which she defines as using an understanding of one's own behavior to help others identify their difficulties
   b. Psychodynamic nursing applies principles of human relations to problems that arise at all levels of human experience
   c. In Peplau's model, the phases of the nurse-patient relationship reflect occurrences in personal interactions
   d. Although separate, these phases overlap and occur over time (see *Changing aspects of the nurse-patient relationship*)
   e. The four phases are orientation, identification, exploitation, and resolution
   f. During these phases, the nurse assumes various roles, such as teacher, resource, counselor, leader, technical expert, and surrogate
2. Orientation
   a. The orientation phase begins when a patient expresses a "felt need"
   b. This need provides the impetus for a meeting between the nurse and the patient
   c. The nurse and the patient meet as strangers and strive to become comfortable with each other while collaboratively defining the problem

CHANGING ASPECTS OF THE NURSE-PATIENT RELATIONSHIP

The nurse and the patient are strangers to each other and may have entirely separate goals and interests.

The roles of each in the problematic situation may differ, partly because of their individual preconceptions about the meaning of the medical problem.

Together, the nurse and the patient can work toward a partially mutual and partially individual understanding of the nature of the medical problem.

Common, shared health goals can result from a mutual understanding of the nature of the problem and of the roles and requirements of the nurse and the patient in solving the problem.

Their collaborative efforts can direct the nurse and the patient toward solving the problem together, productively.

From Peplau, H.E. *Interpersonal Relations in Nursing.* New York: G.P. Putnum & Sons, 1952. Adapted with permission of the author.

d. Collaborative clarifying and defining of the problem allows the patient to direct energy away from the anxiety of unmet needs toward constructive activities

e. The patient and the nurse work together to understand their reactions to each other, mindful of potential influencing factors, such as culture, religion, personal experiences, and preconceived ideas

3. Identification

a. In the identification phase, the patient responds selectively to the people who can meet the patient's defined needs

b. Patient reactions differ; one patient may participate and be interdependent with the nurse, another may be autonomous and independent from the nurse, and yet another may be passive and dependent on the nurse

c. The patient and the nurse must continue to clarify each other's perceptions and expectations because these determine their personal reactions

    d. The nurse's expressed feelings can help an ill patient respond with positive emotions and strengthened personality, which can provide needed satisfaction

    e. During this phase, the patient may begin to feel a sense of belonging and may gain confidence in dealing with the targeted problem

    f. These positive responses can decrease a sense of helplessness and hopelessness, creating an optimistic attitude that further promotes inner strength

4. Exploitation

    a. In the exploitation phase, the patient may use all available services, based on personal interests and needs

    b. The nurse assists the patient in using these services, maintaining a therapeutic relationship at all times

    c. The patient can thereby derive full value from what is offered through the nurse-patient relationship

    d. During this phase, the nurse and the patient can identify new goals; power may shift from the nurse to the patient

    e. The patient may feel like a participant in the helping environment and may develop control over some aspects of the situation

    f. This new outlook may make the patient more demanding, in which case the nurse must use interviewing techniques to explore and understand the patient's actions

5. Resolution

    a. During the resolution phase, after the patient's needs have been met by the collaborative efforts of the nurse and the patient, the therapeutic relationship ends

    b. Resolution is achieved when the patient drifts away from identifying with the nurse and dissolves the nurse-patient bond

    c. Successful resolution results directly from successful completion of the other three phases

    d. The patient moves toward new goals during this phase

C. Peplau's model and the four concepts of the nursing metaparadigm

1. Person

    a. Is defined as an individual; Peplau does not include families, groups, or communities

    b. Is described as a developing organism that strives to reduce anxiety caused by needs

    c. Lives in an unstable equilibrium

2. Environment

    a. Is not specifically defined by Peplau

    b. Is implied in that the nurse must consider culture and values when acclimating the patient to the hospital environment, but Peplau does not address possible environmental influences on the patient

3. Health
   a. Is described as a concept that implies forward movement of personality and other ongoing human processes toward creative, constructive, productive, personal, and community living
   b. Consists of interacting physiologic and interpersonal conditions
   c. Is promoted through the interpersonal process
4. Nursing
   a. Is a significant, therapeutic, interpersonal process that functions cooperatively with other human processes that make health possible
   b. Is a human relationship between an individual who is sick or who has a felt need and a nurse who is educated to recognize and respond to the need for help
   c. Achieves its goal by promoting the patient's development of skills to deal with problems and achieve health; this is a mutual and collaborative process that attempts to resolve the problem
   d. Views the nursing process as having sequential steps that focus on therapeutic interactions
   e. Involves the use of problem-solving techniques by the nurse and patient; according to Peplau, both the nurse and patient learn the problem-solving process from the relationship
   f. Proceeds from the general to the specific in collecting data and clarifying problems, and uses observation, communication, and recording as basic tools

Points to Remember

Peplau's Interpersonal Relations Model has its foundation in the behavioral sciences.

Peplau views her model as evolving from psychodynamic nursing.

The central focus of Peplau's model is the nurse-patient relationship.

The nurse-patient relationship consists of four phases—orientation, identification, exploitation, and resolution.

During these phases, the nurse assumes various roles while interacting with the patient.

Glossary

Health—forward movement of personality and other ongoing human processes in the direction of creative, constructive, productive, personal, and community living

Interpersonal process—interaction between two persons to benefit the person in need

Resource—one of the roles assumed by the nurse during Peplau's phases of interpersonal relations in which the nurse provides specific, necessary information to promote understanding of a problem or new situation

Therapeutic relationship—interpersonal communication between a patient and a nurse to solve the patient's health problems and fulfill personal needs

Henderson's Definition of Nursing

Learning Objectives

After studying this section, the reader should be able to:

- Describe Henderson's Definition of Nursing.

- List the 14 basic needs that figure prominently in Henderson's vision of nursing care.

- Discuss how Henderson addresses the four concepts of the nursing metaparadigm.

IV. Henderson's Definition of Nursing

A. **Introduction**
   1. Virginia Henderson graduated from the Army School of Nursing in 1921
   2. In 1926, she was awarded BS and MA degrees in nursing education from Teachers College, Columbia University, New York City
   3. Her interest in nursing evolved from helping sick and wounded military personnel during World War I
   4. Henderson was motivated to develop her ideas because she had concerns about the function of nurses and the nurse registration laws
      a. She was influenced by her nursing education and practice, her students and colleagues, and nursing leaders of her time
      b. A strong influence was her dislike of the basic nursing education provided by the Army School of Nursing, which emphasized technical competence and mastery of nursing procedures, viewed nursing as an extension of medical practice, and provided no role models
      c. Other influences included her work in psychiatric and pediatric nursing as well as her experiences in community health nursing at the Henry Street Settlement in New York City
   5. In 1955, Henderson first published her Definition of Nursing in a revised version of the textbook *The Principles and Practice of Nursing*
      a. As a result of working on this book, Henderson felt the need to clarify the role of nurses even further
      b. Her involvement as a committee member in a regional National Nursing Council conference also contributed to her need to define nursing
      c. She was also motivated by her dissatisfaction with the 1955 definition of nursing by the American Nurses' Association
   6. In 1966, Henderson clarified her Definition of Nursing in the book *The Nature of Nursing*
      a. She developed her definition based on the sciences of physiology, medicine, psychology, and physics
      b. She acknowledges Ida Orlando as an influence on her concept of the nurse-patient relationship
   7. Henderson has received much recognition, including honorary doctoral degrees, during her career in nursing practice and education; she continues to voice her views on nursing at conferences and on videotape

B. **Definition of Nursing**
   1. General information
      a. Henderson views her work as a philosophical statement rather than a theory because the term *theory* was not used at the time she formulated her ideas
      b. In her definition, Henderson emphasizes the care of both sick and well individuals; she was one of the first theorists to include spiritual aspects of nursing care

    c. According to Henderson, the nurse assists the patient with essential activities to maintain health, recover from illness, or achieve a peaceful death

    d. The patient's independence is an important criterion for health

    e. Henderson identifies 14 basic needs that form the components of nursing care; the nurse helps the patient meet these needs

    f. Henderson's 14 basic needs closely parallel those of Abraham Maslow: 1 to 7 relate to physiology, 8 and 9 relate to safety, 10 relates to self-esteem, 10 and 11 relate to love and belonging, and 11 to 14 relate to self-actualization

    g. Considered together, the 14 basic needs provide a holistic approach to nursing

2. Henderson's basic needs

    a. Breathe normally

    b. Eat and drink adequately

    c. Eliminate body wastes

    d. Move and maintain desirable positions

    e. Sleep and rest

    f. Select suitable clothing

    g. Maintain body temperature

    h. Maintain bodily cleanliness and grooming

    i. Avoid dangers in the environment

    j. Communicate with others to express emotions, needs, fears, or opinions

    k. Worship according to one's faith

    l. Work in a way that provides a sense of accomplishment

    m. Play or participate in various forms of recreation

    n. Learn, discover, or satisfy the curiosity that leads to normal development and health

C. Henderson's definition and the four concepts of the nursing metaparadigm

1. Person

    a. Is viewed by Henderson as an individual requiring assistance to achieve health and independence or a peaceful death; the person and family are viewed as a unit

    b. Is affected by both body and mind

    c. Consists of biological, psychological, sociological, and spiritual components

    d. Is either sick or well and strives toward a state of independence

    e. Has certain basic needs for survival

    f. Needs strength, will, or knowledge to perform activities necessary for healthy living

2. Environment

    a. Is not specifically defined by Henderson

    b. Involves the relationship one shares with one's family

    c. Also involves the community and its responsibility for providing health care; Henderson believes that society wants and expects nurses to provide a service for individuals incapable of functioning independently, but in return she expects society to contribute to nursing education

    d. Can be controlled by healthy individuals; illness may interfere with this ability

    e. Can affect health; personal factors (age, cultural background, physical capacity, and intellect) and physical factors (air, temperature) play a role in a person's well-being

3. Health

    a. Refers to an individual's ability to function independently in relationship to the 14 basic needs

    b. Is a quality of life that is basic to human functioning

    c. Requires strength, will, or knowledge

4. Nursing

    a. Is defined by Henderson as primarily assisting a sick or well individual to perform activities that contribute to health or a peaceful death; the person with sufficient strength, will, or knowledge would perform these activities unaided

    b. Helps a person be independent of assistance as soon as possible or achieve a peaceful death

    c. Requires working interdependently with other members of the health care team; the nurse functions independently of the physician but uses the physician's plan of care to provide holistic care to the patient

    d. Requires basic knowledge of social sciences and humanities; this pioneering belief, which led to baccalaureate education as the basic training for nurses, was not adopted by the American Nurses' Association until 1965

    e. Requires knowledge of social customs and religious practices to assess areas of possible conflict or unmet human needs

    f. Helps a patient meet the 14 basic needs through the formation of a nurse-patient relationship; Henderson identifies three levels of nursing function—substitute (making up for what the patient lacks to be whole), helper (instituting medical interventions), or partner (fostering a therapeutic relationship with the patient and functioning as a member of the health care team)

    g. Is a logical, scientific approach to problem solving that results in individualized care

    h. Involves the use of a written nursing care plan

Points to Remember

Henderson developed her Definition of Nursing because she had concerns about the role and function of nurses.

The nurse's role is to assist an individual who cannot independently perform activities that meet basic needs.

Henderson identifies 14 basic needs of every person.

Individuals need strength, will, and knowledge to perform activities and be healthy.

Henderson advocates the use of a written nursing care plan.

Glossary

Health — state maintained by the patient's ability to function independently

Needs — activities required by an individual for survival

Nursing care plan — measures or activities designed for a patient based on the 14 basic needs and the patient's ability to meet those needs

Abdellah's Typology of Nursing Problems

Learning Objectives
After reading this section, the reader should be able to:

● Describe Abdellah's Typology of Nursing Problems.

● List the 21 nursing problems identified by Abdellah.

● Discuss how Abdellah addresses the four concepts of the nursing metaparadigm.

V. Abdellah's Typology of Nursing Problems

A. Introduction

1. Faye G. Abdellah began her nursing career in 1942 when she received her diploma in nursing from Fitkin Memorial Hospital School of Nursing in Neptune, N.J.
2. In 1945, she received her BS, in 1947 her MA, and in 1955 her EdD from Teachers College, Columbia University, New York City
3. Her varied background includes appointments as chief nurse officer of the United States Public Health Service in 1970 and as concurrent deputy surgeon general in 1982; she retired in 1989
4. Abdellah was motivated to develop her typology by a desire to promote comprehensive, client-centered nursing care
   a. She developed her typology because she realized that nursing needed a strong knowledge base to achieve full professional status and autonomy
   b. She used the problem-solving approach as the basis for her typology
5. Her typology of nursing problems was first published in 1960 in *Patient-Centered Approaches to Nursing*
   a. Abdellah devised her typology from several research studies conducted in the 1950s
   b. In 1973, she refined some of her beliefs about nursing

B. Typology of Nursing Problems

1. General information
   a. The major component of Abdellah's typology is a list of nursing problems, or health care needs of the client
   b. She defines a nursing problem as any condition presented or faced by a client or family for which a nurse can offer assistance
   c. The problem can be *overt* (an apparent condition faced by a client or family) or *covert* (a concealed or hidden condition)
   d. Abdellah described 21 nursing problems subsumed under one of three categories: physical, social, and emotional needs of a client; interpersonal relationships between a nurse and a client; and common elements of client care (see *Abdellah's 21 nursing problems,* page 32)
   e. Abdellah also describes a means of solving a client's problems
2. Problem solving
   a. The analyzer identifies overt and covert problems and interprets, analyzes, and selects an appropriate course of action to solve these problems
   b. Abdellah emphasizes the nurse rather than the client; according to her, a nurse must be able to solve problems to render the best professional nursing care

---

ABDELLAH'S 21 NURSING PROBLEMS

1. Adequate hygiene and physical comfort
2. Optimal activity: exercise, rest, and sleep
3. Safety by preventing accidents, injury, or other trauma and by preventing the spread of infection
4. Good body mechanics and prevention and correction of deformities
5. Adequate oxygen supply to all body cells
6. Nutrition for all body cells
7. Elimination
8. Fluid and electrolyte balance
9. Recognition of the body's physiologic responses to disease (pathological, physiologic, and compensatory)
10. Regulatory mechanisms and functions
11. Sensory function
12. Identification and acceptance of positive and negative expressions, feelings, and reactions
13. Identification and acceptance of the interrelatedness of emotions and organic illness
14. Effective verbal and nonverbal communication
15. Productive interpersonal relationships
16. Progress toward personal spiritual goals
17. A therapeutic environment
18. Awareness of oneself as an individual with varying physical, emotional, and developmental needs
19. Acceptance of the optimum possible goals in light of physical and emotional limitations
20. Community resources as an aid in resolving problems arising from illness
21. Understanding of social problems as influencing factors in illness

From Abdellah et al., *Patient-Centered Approaches to Nursing*. New York: MacMillan Publishing Co., 1960. Adapted with permission of the publisher.

C. **Abdellah's typology and the four concepts of the nursing metaparadigm**
1. Person
   a. Is described by Abdellah as one who has physical, emotional, or sociological needs; helping a person with these needs is nursing's only justification
   b. Is the recipient of nursing care
   c. Includes families as well as individuals
   d. Is capable of learning and of self-help to varying degrees
2. Environment
   a. Is the least discussed concept of Abdellah's typology, although she stated in 1988 that she would have given greater emphasis to environment and health promotion had she been conducting her work today
   b. Includes the atmosphere of a client's room, home, and community; Abdellah also discusses a therapeutic environment but does not define it
3. Health
   a. Is not specifically defined by Abdellah, but she refers to health needs and a healthy state of mind and body; the client's continued health is the purpose of nursing
   b. Is viewed as a state that excludes illness
   c. Can also be described as a state in which the person has no unmet needs and no anticipated or actual impairments

4. Nursing
   a. Is a helping profession
   b. Is a comprehensive service that combines art and science
   c. Does something to or for a client or provides information that helps meet the client's needs, increases or restores self-help ability, or alleviates an impairment
   d. Uses the nursing process, a problem-solving approach
   e. Can use the 21 nursing problems as a guide for nursing care

Points to Remember

Abdellah developed a list of 21 nursing problems, which form the basis for her typology and serve as a guide for nursing care.

Nursing problems can be overt or covert.

The nurse can use the 21 problems as a start-up for the nursing process.

Abdellah views the nursing process as a way to solve client problems.

Glossary

Nursing problem — condition presented or faced by a client or family for which a nurse can offer assistance

Problem solving — process of identifying overt and covert nursing problems and interpreting, analyzing, and selecting appropriate actions to solve these problems

Orlando's Nursing Process Theory

Learning Objectives

After studying this section, the reader should be able to:

● Describe Orlando's Nursing Process Theory.

● Identify the theory's three components.

● Discuss how Orlando addresses the four concepts of the nursing metaparadigm.

VI. Orlando's Nursing Process Theory

A. **Introduction**
   1. Ida Jean Orlando began her nursing career in 1947 after receiving her diploma in nursing from New York Medical College, Flower Fifth Avenue Hospital School of Nursing, New York City
   2. In 1951, she received a BS in public health nursing from St. John's University, New York City, and in 1954, an MA in mental health consultation from Teachers College, Columbia University, New York City
   3. Orlando has held positions in hospital acute care, teaching, research, and clinical consultation
   4. As a research associate at Yale University, she studied the integration of mental health concepts with the basic nursing curriculum
   5. This research led her to publish *The Dynamic Nurse-Patient Relationship: Function, Process, and Principles* (1961), which provides the foundation for her theory
   6. Further research led to the publication of *The Discipline and Teaching of the Nursing Process* in 1972
   7. Orlando conceived her theory from her search for information about the practice of nursing
      a. She attempted to find an organizing principle for professional nursing that makes it a distinct function with a unique focus
      b. She formulated her theory during an era in which the medical model prevailed in health care institutions

B. **Nursing Process Theory**
   1. General information
      a. Orlando's nursing process is based on the manner in which all individuals act
      b. The nursing process is used by a nurse to meet a patient's need for help; meeting this need improves the patient's behavior
      c. This process is also used by other health care workers
      d. The components of Orlando's Nursing Process Theory are patient behavior (Orlando uses the term *patient*), nurse reaction, and nurse action
   2. Patient behavior
      a. The nursing process is set in motion by the patient's behavior
      b. All patient behavior, no matter how insignificant, may represent a cry for help
      c. The patient who cannot resolve a need feels helpless, and the person's behavior reflects this feeling
      d. Patient behavior can be verbal (expressed by language, such as complaints, requests, demands, or refusals) or nonverbal (manifested physiologically, such as heart rate, edema, or motor activity, or vocally, such as crying)

   e. Problems in the nurse-patient relationship can develop if a patient cannot
       communicate a need effectively
3. Nurse reaction
   a. Nurse reaction to a patient's behavior forms the basis for determining
       how a nurse acts; it consists of perception, thought, and feeling
   b. The nurse's first experience with the patient's behavior is through the
       senses; this perception leads to thought, which evokes a feeling
   c. Because these three parts occur automatically and almost simultaneously,
       a nurse must identify each part of the reaction to help the patient
   d. To ensure that the nurse identifies each part of the reaction appropriately,
       Orlando offers three criteria
   e. First, what the nurse says to the patient must match one or all of the
       items contained in the immediate reaction; what the nurse does
       nonverbally must be verbally expressed, and this expression must match
       one or all of the items in the immediate reaction (for instance, the nurse
       might say to the patient, "You look uncomfortable; you are clutching
       your abdomen")
   f. Second, the nurse must clearly communicate to the patient that what the
       nurse says belongs to the nurse's self, not to the patient (for example, "I
       am concerned because you look uncomfortable")
   g. Third, the nurse must ask the patient about the item expressed (the
       communication) to validate or correct it (for instance, "Are you having
       abdominal pain?")
4. Nurse action
   a. Nurse action is whatever the nurse says or does to benefit the patient
   b. It occurs after the nurse interprets the patient's behavior
   c. Nurse action can be *automatic* (decided on for reasons other than the
       patient's immediate need) or *deliberative* (resulting from correctly
       identifying patient needs through validation of an interpretation made
       from the patient's behavior)
   d. Automatic actions include giving medication prescribed by a physician or
       performing routine patient care
   e. Deliberative actions involve exploring the meaning and relevance of an
       action to the patient; these actions are evaluated for effectiveness
       immediately after completion (for example, explaining a procedure to
       relieve the patient's anxiety)
   f. When performing an action, the nurse is influenced by stimuli related to
       the patient's needs (for example, if a patient grimaces in pain, the nurse's
       response is to validate the patient's cry for help and perform a helpful
       action)

C. **Orlando's theory and the four concepts of the nursing metaparadigm**
   1. Person
      a. Is viewed as a human being who exhibits verbal and nonverbal behavior
      b. Has individual needs and abilities to deal with situations

2. Environment
   a. Is not specifically defined by Orlando
   b. Is implied in the nursing situation that occurs between a nurse and a patient; Orlando addresses the nursing system in institutions but does not discuss how a patient or a nurse's action is affected by the environment
3. Health
   a. Is not specifically defined by Orlando
   b. Can be inferred from her theory as a feeling of adequacy and well-being and freedom from mental or physical discomfort
   c. Is a sense of comfort
4. Nursing
   a. Is a distinct profession that functions autonomously
   b. Concerns itself with an individual's real or potential need for help in an immediate situation
   c. Uses the nursing process (nurse-patient interaction) to relieve a patient's feelings of helplessness or suffering
   d. Attempts to relieve a patient's mental or physical discomfort and not add to patient distress
   e. Tries to enhance a patient's sense of well-being and improve behavior and self-care abilities
   f. Views the patient holistically
   g. Is dynamic and responsive to changes in a patient's situation
   h. Involves a continuous exchange of information and action; it is triggered by patient behavior, which leads to nurse reaction, then to nurse action, and back to patient behavior

Points to Remember

Orlando's theory has three components — patient behavior, nurse reaction (interpretation of the patient's behavior), and nurse action.

The patient's behavior is an expression of need and can be verbal or nonverbal.

According to Orlando's theory, the nursing process is triggered by a patient's behavior.

The nurse's action is based on interpretation of the patient's behavior and can be automatic or deliberate.

Glossary

Deliberative action — nursing action designed to identify and meet a patient's need

Nurse reaction — second component of Orlando's theory, which encompasses perception, thought, and feeling (interpretation of patient behavior)

Patient behavior — verbal or nonverbal actions of the patient that reflect a need for help

Hall's Core, Care, and Cure Model

Learning Objectives

After studying this section, the reader should be able to:

- Describe Hall's Core, Care, and Cure Model.

- Identify components of the three circles in this model.

- Discuss how Hall addresses the four concepts of the nursing metaparadigm.

VII. Hall's Core, Care, and Cure Model

A. **Introduction**
   1. Lydia Hall received her diploma in nursing from York (Pa.) Hospital School of Nursing
   2. She earned a BS in public health nursing and an MA in natural sciences from Teachers College, Columbia University, New York City
   3. Her background includes positions in education, consultation, and nursing practice
   4. In 1963, she developed and designed the Loeb Center for Nursing and Rehabilitation at Montefiore Hospital in New York City
      a. This center was founded on her beliefs about nursing care and her concern for education
      b. According to Hall, the need for professional nursing care increases as the need for medical care decreases; professional nursing care can expedite patient recovery
      c. The success of the center provided empirical evidence to support her beliefs
   5. She served as administrative director of the Loeb Center until her death in 1969
   6. Hall based her model on the behavioral sciences
      a. She drew extensively from psychology and psychiatry
      b. She was strongly influenced by Carl Rogers's work in patient-centered therapy and his views on being a person
   7. She published information about her model in numerous nursing journals in the mid- to late-1960s

B. **Core, Care, and Cure Model**
   1. General information
      a. Hall's nursing model provides a basis for nursing care
      b. She formulated her model at a time when health care was dominated by the practice of medicine; her ideas of nurses controlling nursing care were considered revolutionary
      c. Her model consists of three interlocking circles—the core circle, the care circle, and the cure circle—each of which represents a specific aspect of nursing (See *Core, care, and cure model*, page 43)
      d. According to Hall, nursing functions are different in each circle
      e. The circles are interrelated to emphasize the importance of a whole person approach
      f. The size and importance of the circles change in relation to a patient's progress
   2. The core circle
      a. Refers to the patient
      b. Includes nursing care that revolves around a nurse's therapeutic use of self

      c. Involves developing an interpersonal relationship with a patient, which allows the patient to express feelings about disease and furthers patient maturity and self-identity

      d. Is shared by the nurse with psychologists, psychiatrists, social workers, and members of the clergy

3. The care circle

      a. Refers to the patient's body

      b. Represents the nurturing aspect of nursing care

      c. Involves intimate body care, such as bathing and feeding; a nurse uses knowledge of the natural and biological sciences as a basis for this care

      d. Is exclusive to nursing; a nurse is in charge of care

      e. Includes teaching, which improves the patient's core

4. The cure circle

      a. Refers to pathological processes or the disease

      b. Involves helping a patient and family members through the medical, surgical, and rehabilitative measures instituted by the physician

      c. Includes an active role as patient advocate; from the patient's viewpoint, the nurse's role in the cure circle may take on the negative quality of avoiding pain rather than the positive quality of providing comfort

      d. Is shared with the physician

C. Hall's model and the four concepts of the nursing metaparadigm

1. Person

      a. Is not specifically defined by Hall

      b. Is composed of three parts: person (core circle), body (care circle), and pathology (cure circle)

      c. Learns how to achieve maximum potential; a patient gets to the "core" through learning

      d. Is the source for self-healing; a nurse provides the necessary care and support

      e. Behaves according to personal feelings and not knowledge

      f. Is unique and capable of learning and growth

2. Environment

      a. Is discussed but not specifically defined by Hall

      b. Must be conducive to self-development; Hall's belief that the hospital environment was inadequate led her to found the Loeb Center

      c. Is secondary to the person; any nursing actions taken in relation to the environment should assist the patient in attaining a personal goal

3. Health

      a. Is not specifically defined by Hall, although she does describe illness as a behavior directed by a person's feelings of self-awareness

      b. Can be inferred as a state of self-awareness; a person consciously selects behaviors that are personally beneficial

      c. Involves helping a patient examine self-behavior to identify and overcome problems and develop self-identity and maturity

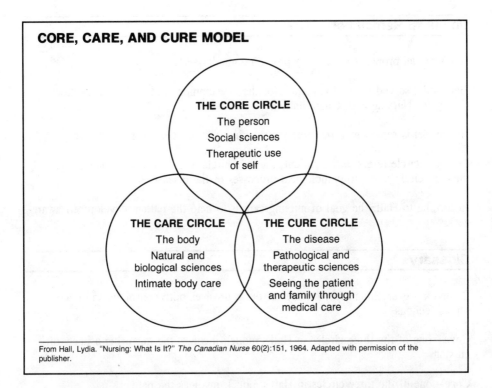

CORE, CARE, AND CURE MODEL

THE CORE CIRCLE
The person
Social sciences
Therapeutic use
of self

THE CARE CIRCLE
The body
Natural and
biological sciences
Intimate body care

THE CURE CIRCLE
The disease
Pathological and
therapeutic sciences
Seeing the patient
and family through
medical care

From Hall, Lydia. "Nursing: What Is It?" *The Canadian Nurse* 60(2):151, 1964. Adapted with permission of the publisher.

4. Nursing
   a. Is a profession that involves nurturing and comforting; according to Hall, a patient should receive care only from professional nurses who can take complete responsibility for the care
   b. Involves interacting with a patient in a complex process of teaching and learning
   c. Strives to form a relationship that helps the patient develop self-identity
   d. Combines knowledge of medical procedures and diseases with teaching and learning skills to provide the patient with individualized care
   e. Requires participation in the core, care, and cure circles

Points to Remember

Hall's model proposes a basis for providing nursing care.

Her model served as the foundation for the development and design of the Loeb Center for Nursing and Rehabilitation.

Her model is represented by three interlocking circles — core, care, and cure.

The core circle refers to the patient, the care circle refers to the patient's body, and the cure circle refers to pathological processes or the disease.

According to Hall, the goal of nursing care is to help the patient develop self-awareness.

Glossary

Behavior — everything a person says or does; involves both conscious and unconscious feelings

Care — one of the three circles in Hall's model; involves the nurturing aspects of nursing

Core — one of the three circles in Hall's model; involves the patient

Cure — one of the three circles in Hall's model; involves the disease or pathology and the patient

Professional nursing — care given by nurses who are educated in the behavioral sciences and who can take responsibility for and deliver coordinated care to the patient

Therapeutic use of self — use of reflection as a communication technique in which seminal ideas or issues are raised repeatedly by the nurse, encouraging further exploration of the patient's feelings

Wiedenbach's Helping Art of Clinical Nursing Theory

Learning Objectives

After studying this section, the reader should be able to:

● Describe Wiedenbach's Helping Art of Clinical Nursing Theory.

● Identify the three components of this prescriptive theory.

● Identify the three components of nursing practice.

● Discuss how Wiedenbach addresses the four concepts of the nursing metaparadigm.

VIII. Wiedenbach's Helping Art of Clinical Nursing Theory

A. **Introduction**
   1. Ernestine Wiedenbach began her nursing career in 1925 after receiving her diploma in nursing from The Johns Hopkins School of Nursing, Baltimore
   2. In 1922, she had graduated from Wellesley (Mass.) College with a liberal arts degree
   3. Wiedenbach received her master's degree in public health nursing from Teachers College, Columbia University, New York City, in 1934 and was certified in nurse midwifery by the Maternity Center Association in New York City in 1946
   4. She has held positions in nursing practice and education and has published many articles about nursing
   5. Wiedenbach became interested in nursing as a child and used many sources in developing her theory
      a. She was influenced by fellow faculty members, including Ida Orlando, Patricia James, and James Dickoff
      b. She also drew from her extensive experience in clinical practice and teaching
   6. Wiedenbach first published her ideas in 1964 in *Clinical Nursing: A Helping Art*
   7. She further refined her theory in "Nurses' Wisdom in Nursing Theory," published in 1970 by the *American Journal of Nursing*

B. **Helping Art of Clinical Nursing Theory**
   1. General information
      a. Wiedenbach proposes a prescriptive theory for nursing, which is described as a conceiving of a desired situation and the ways to attain it
      b. Prescriptive theory directs action toward an explicit goal
      c. It consists of three factors: central purpose, prescription, and realities
      d. A nurse develops a prescription based on a central purpose and implements it according to the realities of the situation
   2. Central purpose
      a. Purpose refers to what the nurse wants to accomplish
      b. It is the overall goal toward which a nurse strives; it transcends the immediate intent of the assignment or task by specifically directing activities toward the patient's good
      c. It is based on the nurse's personal philosophy — an attitude toward life and reality that evolves from specific beliefs and a code of conduct
      d. A nurse's philosophy is unique and personal; it motivates action, guides thinking, and influences decisions
      e. The three essential components of a nursing philosophy are a reverence for life; a respect for the dignity, worth, autonomy, and individuality of each person; and a resolve to act dynamically based on one's beliefs
   3. Prescription
      a. Prescription refers to the plan of care for a patient

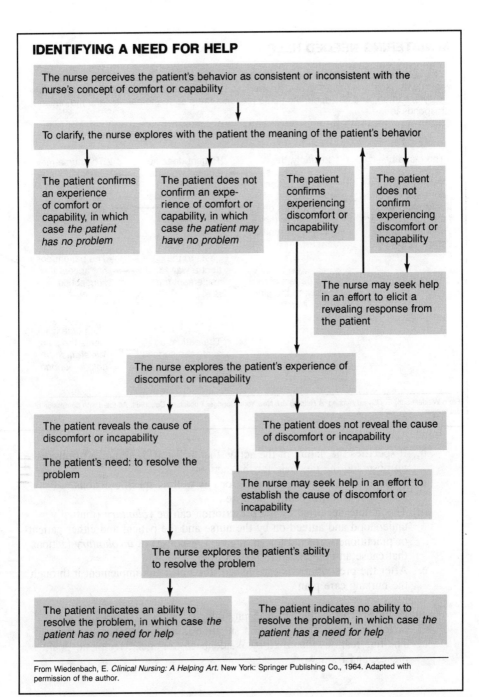

IDENTIFYING A NEED FOR HELP

The nurse perceives the patient's behavior as consistent or inconsistent with the nurse's concept of comfort or capability

To clarify, the nurse explores with the patient the meaning of the patient's behavior

The patient confirms an experience of comfort or capability, in which case *the patient has no problem*

The patient does not confirm an experience of comfort or capability, in which case *the patient may have no problem*

The patient confirms experiencing discomfort or incapability

The patient does not confirm experiencing discomfort or incapability

The nurse may seek help in an effort to elicit a revealing response from the patient

The nurse explores the patient's experience of discomfort or incapability

The patient reveals the cause of discomfort or incapability

The patient's need: to resolve the problem

The patient does not reveal the cause of discomfort or incapability

The nurse may seek help in an effort to establish the cause of discomfort or incapability

The nurse explores the patient's ability to resolve the problem

The patient indicates an ability to resolve the problem, in which case *the patient has no need for help*

The patient indicates no ability to resolve the problem, in which case *the patient has a need for help*

From Wiedenbach, E. *Clinical Nursing: A Helping Art.* New York: Springer Publishing Co., 1964. Adapted with permission of the author.

MINISTERING NEEDED HELP

The nurse formulates a plan for meeting the patient's need for help based on available resources: what the patient thinks, knows, can do, and has done plus what the nurse thinks, knows, can do, and has done; the nurse presents the plan to the patient, and the patient responds to it

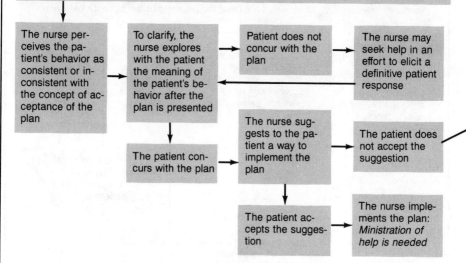

From Wiedenbach, E. *Clinical Nursing: A Helping Art.* New York: Springer Publishing Co., 1964. Adapted with permission of the author.

    b. It specifies the nature of the action that will fulfill the nurse's central purpose and the rationale for that action

    c. It may indicate broad general actions as well as specific actions congruent with the central purpose

    d. The actions specified by the prescription can be *voluntary* (mutually understood and agreed on by the nurse and the patient and either patient- or practitioner-directed for an intended response) or *involuntary* (actions that cause an unintended response)

    e. After the prescription is established, the nurse can implement it through the nursing care plan

4. Realities

    a. Realities refer to the physical, physiologic, emotional, and spiritual factors that come into play in a situation involving nursing actions

    b. The five realities identified by Weidenbach are agent, recipient, goal, means, and framework

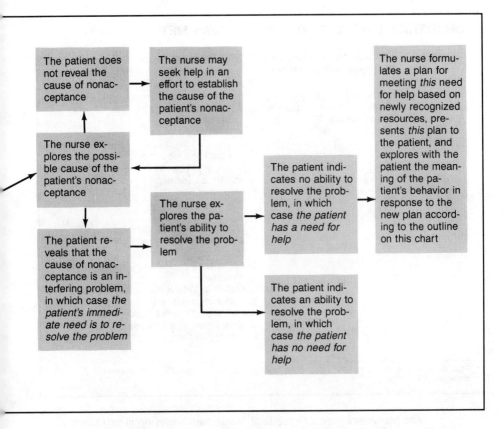

c. The *agent* is the practicing nurse or a designee who has the personal attributes, capacities, capabilities, commitment, and competence to provide nursing care

d. As the agent, a nurse directs all actions toward the goal

e. The *recipient* is the patient who has personal attributes, problems, capabilities, aspirations, and abilities to cope

f. The recipient is the one who receives a nurse's actions or on whose behalf actions are taken; the recipient is vulnerable and dependent

g. The *goal* is the nurse's desired outcome; it directs actions and suggests the reasons for taking those actions

h. The *means* are the activities and devices used by the nurse to achieve the goal

i. They include specific skills, procedures, and techniques; the manner in which a nurse uses these means relates to the central purpose and prescription

VALIDATING THAT A NEED FOR HELP WAS MET

The nurse perceives the patient's behavior as consistent or inconsistent with the nurse's concept of comfort or capability

To clarify, the nurse explores with the patient the meaning of the patient's behavior

The patient provides convincing evidence of comfort or capability, in which case *the need for help has been met*

The patient does not provide convincing evidence of comfort or capability, in which case *the need for help may not have been met*

The nurse may need to reconstruct experience with the patient to ascertain:
- whether the need for help has been identified
- whether the nurse has met the need in an acceptable way
- whether the nurse needs help to know where to start again and take appropriate action

From Wiedenbach, E. *Clinical Nursing: A Helping Art*. New York: Springer Publishing Co., 1964. Adapted with permission of the author.

    j. The *framework* refers to the facilities in which nursing is practiced; it comprises human, environmental, professional, and organizational aspects of care

C. Nursing practice
  1. General information
    a. Wiedenbach views nursing as an art based on goal-directed care
    b. Factual and speculative knowledge, judgment, and skills are necessary for effective nursing practice
    c. Wiedenbach's vision of nursing practice closely parallels the assessment, implementation, and evaluation steps of the nursing process
    d. In addition, she identifies seven levels of awareness: *sensation* (reception of stimulus), *perception* (reaction to how stimulus is viewed), *assumption* (overview of the stimulus and the situation), *realization* (gathering of resources to control actions), *insight* (use of reason to gain more information about the situation), *design* (formulation of a plan), and *decision* (action that furthers the plan)

      e. According to Wiedenbach, nursing practice consists of identifying a patient's need for help, ministering the needed help, and validating that the need for help was met

2. Identification

      a. Involves viewing the patient as an individual with unique experiences and understanding the patient's perception of the condition

      b. Determines a patient's need for help based on the existence of a need, whether the patient realizes the need, what prevents the patient from meeting the need, and whether the patient cannot meet the need alone (see *Identifying a need for help,* page 47)

3. Ministration

      a. Refers to provision of needed help

      b. Requires an identified need and a patient who wants help (see *Ministering needed help,* pages 48 and 49)

4. Validation

      a. Refers to a collection of evidence that shows a patient's needs have been met and that his functional ability has been restored as a direct result of the nurse's actions

      b. Is based on patient-oriented evidence (see *Validating that a need for help was met*)

D. Wiedenbach's theory and the four concepts of the nursing metaparadigm

1. Person

      a. Is a human being

      b. Is endowed with the unique potential to develop internal resources to maintain and sustain the self

      c. Strives toward self-direction and independence

      d. Desires to make the best use of personal abilities and to fulfill responsibilities; any action represents the person's best judgment at that moment

      e. Relies on self-awareness and self-acceptance to maintain a sense of integrity and self-worth

2. Environment

      a. Is not specifically defined by Wiedenbach

      b. Is addressed in the realities component of her prescriptive theory (factors in realities constitute a dynamic conglomerate of ideas, events, experiences, and objects in contact with a patient)

3. Health

      a. Is not specifically defined by Wiedenbach

      b. Is addressed in her discussion of the nurse-patient relationship and the need for help

4. Nursing

      a. Is described by Wiedenbach as a clinical practice discipline implemented for a desired result; the nurse is described as one who acts, thinks, and feels and whose actions are based on the ability to think and feel

      b. Helps a patient overcome difficulties and meet the need for help

c. Uses factual, speculative, and practical knowledge, judgment, and procedural and communication skills

d. Is an art that uses individualized actions carried out by the nurse in a one-to-one relationship with the patient

e. Involves three operations: stimulus (the patient's behavior), preconception (idea of what the patient might be like), and interpretation (comparison between the nurse's perception of the patient's behavior and the nurse's prior expectations of the behavior); these operations form the basis for a nurse's reactions

Points to Remember

Wiedenbach offers a prescriptive theory for nursing.

The three components of her prescriptive theory are central purpose, prescription, and realities.

According to Wiedenbach, a nurse's central purpose is based on a personal philosophy.

The three essential aspects of a nursing philosophy are a reverence for life, a respect for the dignity of each person, and a resolve to act dynamically in relation to one's beliefs.

Wiedenbach also offers a conceptualization of nursing practice that includes identifying a patient's need for help, ministering the help needed, and validating that the action taken was helpful to the patient.

Glossary

Factual knowledge — that which has been proved to be true

Realization — one of the seven levels of Wiedenbach's nursing process in which the nurse begins to validate assumptions about the patient's behavior

Skills — deliberate acts carried out for a specific purpose and characterized by harmony, precision, and proficiency

Speculative knowledge — theories and general principles that seek to explain phenomena, beliefs, or concepts

Levine's Conservation Model

Learning Objectives

After studying this section, the reader should be able to:

- Describe Levine's Conservation Model.

- Identify the four conservation principles.

- Identify the four levels of holistic response.

- Discuss how Levine's model addresses the four concepts of the nursing metaparadigm.

IX. Levine's Conservation Model

A. **Introduction**
1. Myra E. Levine received her diploma in nursing in 1944 from Cook County School of Nursing, Chicago
2. In 1949, she received her BS in nursing from the University of Chicago, and in 1962, her MS in nursing from Wayne State University, Detroit
3. Levine has held positions as staff nurse, administrator, teacher, supervisor, clinical instructor, and director of nursing services
4. She developed her model as a starting point for theory development
   a. She planned to separate the realms of nursing and medicine and explain why nurses perform activities
   b. She used general systems theory, Hans Selye's stress theory, Erik Erickson's developmental theory, and the work of such nursing theorists as Florence Nightingale, Martha Rogers, and Faye Abdellah
5. Levine first published her model in "Adaptation and Assessment: A Rationale for Nursing Intervention" in the *American Journal of Nursing* in 1966
   a. This article was followed by two additional articles that refined the model's components
   b. In 1969, she presented a comprehensive description of her model in *Introduction to Clinical Nursing*
   c. In 1971, 1973, and 1978, Levine published further refinements of her model
   d. In 1988, she published the most recent version of her work in *Conceptual Models for Nursing Practice*
6. Levine's Conservation Model, which addresses total patient care, has two components – the conservation principles and the organismic response, or pursuit of wholeness
   a. Her model is limited to persons already in a state of illness
   b. She focuses on the nursing interventions used during the patient's adaptation and response to illness; these actions are aimed at restoring the patient's wholeness, integrity, and well-being

B. **Conservation principles**
1. General information
   a. Levine bases her model on nursing intervention as a conservation activity that maintains a person's wholeness or totality
   b. She uses four conservation principles to explain all nursing interventions that maintain a patient's health
   c. These principles attempt to provide a scientific basis for nursing actions
2. Conservation of energy
   a. Refers to an individual's need for a balance of energy and a constant renewal of energy resources
   b. Involves balancing energy output with energy input to improve health

3. Conservation of structural integrity
   a. Refers to an individual's need for healing, or maintaining and restoring the body's elements
   b. Involves preventing physical breakdown and promoting healing
4. Conservation of personal integrity
   a. Refers to an individual's need to maintain and restore self-identity and self-worth
   b. Involves acknowledging a person's uniqueness and identity, such as calling a patient by name or respecting personal privacy
5. Conservation of social integrity
   a. Refers to an individual's need for interaction with others as a social being
   b. Involves recognizing the importance of human interaction, including that of the patient with significant others
6. Importance of social integrity
   a. According to Levine, health is socially determined
   b. Individual coping patterns, such as adapting to a crisis, determine social acceptance

C. **Organismic response**
   1. General information
      a. To survive, a person must adapt to the environment
      b. Individuals can choose several ways of adapting to the environment; this is called *redundancy*
      c. The levels of redundant choices are part of the person's organismic response; some responses are immediate, whereas others are long-term
      d. Levine identifies four levels of organismic response: fight or flight response, inflammatory response, response to stress, and sensory response
   2. Fight or flight response
      a. Is the most primitive response to a real or perceived threat
      b. Causes the individual either to stay and face the threat or to run from it
   3. Inflammatory response
      a. Is a mechanism that protects a person from a hostile environment
      b. Maintains the body's structural integrity and promotes healing
   4. Response to stress
      a. Is a nonspecific bodily response in which all systems within the individual adapt (for example, the psychological and social responses to limb amputation)
      b. Is based on Hans Selye's stress theory, or general adaptation syndrome
   5. Sensory response
      a. Is based on a person's perceptual awareness; causes use of the senses
      b. Is used to gather information from the environment for self-protection

D. Levine's model and the four concepts of the nursing metaparadigm
1. Person
   a. Is viewed by Levine as a holistic individual or open system
   b. Can be distinguished from a nursing patient: according to Levine, a *person* is an everchanging organism in constant interaction with the environment and striving to maintain integrity, whereas a *nursing patient* is a whole person in need of assistance to conserve energy and maintain structural, personal, or social integrity
   c. Experiences orderly, sequential change through adaptation; health and illness are patterns of adaptive change
   d. Survives by using one of the four organismic responses
2. Environment
   a. Is *internal* (within a person, such as the body's response to bacteria)
   b. Is *external* (consisting of three parts: *perceptual environment,* to which a person responds by using the five senses — sight, sound, smell, taste, and touch; *operational environment,* such as pollutants or radiation, to which a person responds physically; and *conceptual environment,* including past experiences and future ideas, to which a person responds through traditions, beliefs, or values)
   c. Includes the nurse
3. Health
   a. Is described by Levine as a pattern of adaptation or change and is viewed as a continuum
   b. Involves adapting by degrees — that is, gradually rather than by extremes
   c. Maintains a person's unity and integrity
4. Nursing
   a. Is a discipline based on the dependence of people and their relationships with others
   b. Involves human interaction to promote the wholeness of a dependent person and to assist the person in adapting to a state of health
   c. Requires skills and scientific knowledge when interacting with a patient
   d. Entails active participation in every aspect of a patient's internal and external environment
   e. Uses each of the conservation principles to identify areas of intervention
   f. Consists of observing the patient, planning and performing appropriate interventions, and evaluating their effectiveness
   g. Assumes that the nurse and the patient participate together in the patient's care
   h. Recommends trophicognosis as an alternative to nursing diagnosis
   i. Focuses on only one patient at a time and concentrates on the present, with the patient in an altered state of health

Points to Remember

Levine's model is based on four conservation principles — conservation of energy, structural integrity, personal integrity, and social integrity.

Levine focuses on nursing interventions that promote a patient's adaptation and response to illness.

The patient's environment includes both internal and external aspects.

The nurse is considered part of the patient's environment.

According to Levine's model, the patient is in a dependent state.

Glossary

Adaptation — adjustment to the environment that is accomplished with the least expenditure of effort and resources

Organismic response — ability of an organism (including a patient) to adapt to the environment

Trophicognosis — method of ascribing nursing care needs to address a patient deficit in one of the four conservation principles; Levine's term for "nursing diagnosis"

Johnson's Behavioral Systems Model

Learning Objectives

After studying this section, the reader should be able to:

- Describe Johnson's Behavioral Systems Model.

- Identify the seven subsystems of the model.

- Discuss how Johnson addresses the four concepts of the nursing metaparadigm.

X. Johnson's Behavioral Systems Model

A. **Introduction**
1. Dorothy E. Johnson received her associate degree in arts from Armstrong Junior College, Savannah, Georgia, in 1938
2. In 1942, she received her BS in nursing from Vanderbilt University, Nashville, Tenn., and in 1948, her MS in public health from Harvard University, Boston
3. She began writing soon after completing her undergraduate program and continued during her teaching career at the University of California, Los Angeles
4. Most of her professional experience is in teaching (she was a mentor to Sister Callista Roy), but her background also includes positions as staff nurse and advisor to schools of nursing
5. Johnson first proposed her model in 1968 to foster the "efficient and effective behavioral functioning in the patient to prevent illness"
   a. During the 1970s, other nurses, notably Sister Callista Roy and Joan Riehl-Sisca, based their conceptualizations of nursing on Johnson's model
   b. In 1980, Johnson published her Behavioral Systems Model in *Conceptual Models for Nursing Practice*
6. Johnson based her model on Florence Nightingale's belief that nursing is designed to help people prevent or recover from illness or injury
   a. She borrowed ideas from systems theory to explain that nursing is concerned with the individual as an integrated whole
   b. She developed her model from the works of researchers in psychology, sociology, and ethnology

B. **Behavioral subsystems**
1. General information
   a. Johnson's model views the person as a *behavioral system* comprised of a set of organized, interactive, interdependent, and integrated subsystems
   b. The system maintains constancy through actions and behaviors that are regulated and controlled by biological, psychological, and sociological factors
   c. The behavioral system continually strives to maintain a steady state by adjusting and adapting to internal and external forces
   d. Each behavioral subsystem has *structural requirements* (goal, predisposition to act, scope of action, and behavior) and *functional requirements* (protection from harmful influences, nurturance, and stimulation to enhance growth and prevent stagnation)
   e. To ensure growth and development, these requirements must be met by the person alone or through outside assistance
   f. Johnson identifies seven subsystems that carry out special functions for the system as a whole
2. Affiliative subsystem
   a. Is the first to develop in an individual

    b. Forms the basis for all social organization
    c. Promotes survival and provides a sense of security
    d. Results in social inclusion, intimacy, and the formation of strong social bonds

3. Dependency subsystem
    a. Promotes helping or nurturing behavior from others
    b. Closely parallels the affiliative subsystem
    c. Results in approval, attention, recognition, and physical assistance

4. Ingestive subsystem
    a. Involves food intake
    b. Relates to the biological need for food and the psychological meanings and structures of social events surrounding food consumption
    c. Results in appetite satisfaction

5. Eliminative subsystem
    a. Involves behaviors surrounding the excretion of waste from the body
    b. Includes the psychological meanings and structures of socially acceptable behaviors for waste elimination
    c. Is based on learned behaviors

6. Sexual subsystem
    a. Involves behaviors associated with procreation and sexual gratification
    b. Includes psychologically and socially acceptable behaviors, such as courtship and mating
    c. Results in the development of sex role identity and sex role behavior

7. Aggressive subsystem
    a. Involves behaviors related to self-protection and preservation of the self and society
    b. Includes the belief that aggression is learned and harmful and that people and property must be respected and protected
    c. Includes acknowledgment of real or imaginary dangers to develop defenses to these threats

8. Achievement subsystem
    a. Involves behaviors related to manipulation of the environment to gain mastery and control over some aspect of oneself or environment; this control is measured against a standard of excellence
    b. Includes intellectual, physical, creative, mechanical, and social skills

C. Johnson's model and the four concepts of the nursing metaparadigm
1. Person
    a. Is an open, interrelated system identified by actions and behaviors that are regulated and controlled by biological, psychological, and sociological factors
    b. Continually strives to maintain a steady state by adapting and adjusting to environmental forces that cause an imbalance; when an imbalance, or health problem, occurs, the person's physical, social, or psychological integrity is threatened

    c. Is an individual composed of seven open and interactive subsystems; a disturbance in one usually affects the others

    d. Is unique, possessing an individual and distinguishing set of behaviors

2. Environment

    a. Is not specifically defined by Johnson; she refers to a person's internal and external environment but does not explain what they are

    b. Interacts with the person

3. Health

    a. Is defined as balance and stability of a person's behavioral system; instability, or illness, is not addressed directly but can be inferred as a malfunction of the behavioral system

    b. Is demonstrated by orderly, purposeful, predictable behavior that effectively and efficiently manages a person's relationship to the environment

4. Nursing

    a. Views the patient as a behavioral system

    b. Is an external regulatory force that acts to preserve optimal organization and integration of a patient's behavior when the patient encounters a threat to physical or social health

    c. Is indicated only when a system becomes unstable; the goal of nursing is to maintain or restore behavioral system balance and stability and integrated subsystem functioning

    d. Uses outside regulatory control mechanisms, such as teaching, setting limits on behavior, and providing needed environmental resources

    e. Requires a strong background in the physical and social sciences

Points to Remember

Johnson's Behavioral Systems Model advocates fostering efficient and effective behavioral functioning in a patient.

The patient is a behavioral system composed of seven subsystems.

An imbalance in any subsystem results in disequilibrium.

Each subsystem has functional and structural requirements.

The nurse intervenes to restore, maintain, or attain behavioral system balance and stability at the highest possible level for the individual.

Glossary

Equilibrium — stability or balance of all subsystems in the patient's behavioral system

Functional requirements — characteristics of each subsystem that must be maintained for balance, including protection, stimulation, and nurturance

Structural requirements — characteristics of each subsystem that must be maintained for balance, including its goal, predisposition to act, scope of action, and behavior

Rogers's Unitary Human Beings Model

Learning Objectives
After studying this section, the reader should be able to:

● Identify the four building blocks of Rogers's Unitary Human Beings Model.

● Describe the three Principles of Homeodynamics.

● Discuss how Rogers addresses the four concepts of the nursing metaparadigm.

XI. Rogers's Unitary Human Beings Model

A. **Introduction**
  1. Martha Rogers began her nursing career after receiving a diploma in nursing from Knoxville (Tenn.) General Hospital School of Nursing in 1936
  2. In 1937, she received her BS in public health nursing from George Peabody College, Nashville, Tenn., and in 1945, her MA in public health nursing supervision from Teachers College, Columbia University, New York City
  3. In 1952, she earned an MPH, and in 1954, a ScD from Johns Hopkins University, Baltimore
  4. Rogers has held numerous staff and leadership positions in community health nursing, education, and research
  5. In 1970, she presented her model for the first time in *An Introduction to the Theoretical Basis of Nursing*
  6. Over the years, Rogers continued to clarify her ideas by adding, redefining, changing, or removing principles
  7. In 1980, she developed the Science of Unitary Man Model; in 1983, the Science of Unitary Human Beings Model; and in 1986, the Dimensions of Health: A View from Space
  8. Rogers was prompted to develop her model because of the need for nursing to have a distinct and unique body of knowledge
     a. Rogers drew from her background in the liberal arts and sciences
     b. She also used sources from anthropology, psychology, sociology, astronomy, religion, philosophy, history, biology, physics, mathematics, and literature
     c. She developed the model using a deductive approach
  9. Rogers's model is closely related to the general systems theory

B. **Unitary Human Beings Model**
  1. General information
     a. Rogers's model is based on her assumptions about the person and interaction with the environment
     b. She uses four building blocks to develop her model: energy fields, universe of open systems, pattern, and four dimensionality
     c. *Energy fields* are the fundamental units of both living and nonliving things; they are unique, dynamic, open, and infinite
     d. Rogers identifies two energy fields: the human field (unitary man) and the environmental field
     e. *Universe of open systems* refers to the idea that energy fields are open, infinite, and interactive (integral)
     f. *Pattern* is the characteristic of an energy field; it is perceived as a wave that changes continuously, becoming increasingly complex and diverse
     g. The pattern and organization of an energy field are manifested by its observable properties, such as human behavior

h. *Four dimensionality* refers to a nonlinear domain without spatial or temporal attributes; its boundaries are imaginary and continuously fluctuating
i. The Principles of Homeodynamics are derived from these four building blocks

2. Principles of Homeodynamics
   a. Rogers views homeodynamics as a means of understanding life and the mechanisms that affect it
   b. According to Rogers, homeodynamics can provide a nurse with knowledge of how to intervene to redirect a client in a desired direction
   c. These principles have evolved from Rogers's original work to her current model
   d. In *An Introduction to the Theoretical Basis for Nursing* (1970), Rogers identified four Principles of Homeodynamics: resonancy, helicy, reciprocity (continuous and mutual interaction between human and environmental fields), and synchrony (simultaneous change in human and environmental fields at a specific point)
   e. In *Nursing: A Science of Unitary Man* (1980), she replaced reciprocity and synchrony with complimentarity (continuous, mutual, and simultaneous interaction between human and environmental fields)
   f. In *Science of Unitary Human Beings* (1983) and her current model, *Dimensions of Health: A View from Space* (1986), she replaced complimentarity with integrality

3. Integrality
   a. Integrality refers to the continuous and mutual interaction between the human and environmental fields
   b. Because the two fields are inseparable, both have the same features
   c. As a result, sequential changes in life processes take place at the same time and in the same manner in both fields
   d. These life process changes occur as continuous revisions

4. Resonancy
   a. Resonancy refers to the continuous change from lower-frequency (longer) to higher-frequency (shorter) wave patterns in the human and environmental fields
   b. It describes the nature of the change that occurs between the two energy fields
   c. Life process changes are depicted as rhythmical vibrations oscillating at various frequencies and at varying intensities
   d. The continuous change from lower to higher frequencies indicates movement toward increasing complexity of the field

5. Helicy
   a. Helicy refers to the continuous, probabilistic, increasing diversity of the human and environmental fields; it is characterized by nonrepeating *rhythmicities*
   b. It describes the nature and direction of change occurring in the energy fields

   c. Helicy is viewed as change occurring along a spiraling, longitudinal axis bound by space and time
   d. The human field becomes increasingly diverse over time, as it incorporates past patterns and develops new ones
   e. As a person ages, old patterns are not repeated but can recur at more complex levels
   f. Changes in the life process are irreversible; thus the human and environmental fields are repatterned

C. **Rogers's model and the four concepts of the nursing metaparadigm**
   1. Person
      a. Is described as an organized energy field with a unique pattern
      b. Is viewed as a unified whole (unitary man) possessing integrity and manifesting characteristics more than and different from the sum of the parts
      c. Continuously exchanges matter and energy with the environmental field, resulting in life process changes
      d. Experiences a continuous repatterning from interaction with the environment; repatterning evolves irreversibly and unidirectionally along space and time, resulting in an increasingly complex and innovative person
      e. Is identified by his pattern and organization, which reflects his wholeness
      f. Has the capacity for abstraction and imagery, language and thought, sensation and emotion; he can participate creatively in change
      g. Lives in a universe subject to the laws of probability, which provide a basis for predictions, a necessary component for intervention
   2. Environment
      a. Is described as an irreducible four-dimensional energy field identified by pattern and having characteristics different from those of its parts
      b. Is considered to be all that is external to unitary man; a specific environmental field exists for each human field
      c. Is an open system
      d. Is infinite; environmental change is continuous, creative, probabilistic, and mutual with the human field and is characterized by increasing diversity and complexity
      e. Is identified by continuously changing wave patterns
   3. Health
      a. Is not clearly defined by Rogers
      b. Is used to describe wellness and the absence of disease and major illness; Rogers uses the terms *health* and *illness* to identify patterns that denote behaviors of high or low value, the value being determined by the individual and subject to change based on the individual's behavior
   4. Nursing
      a. Is an art and science that seeks to study the nature and direction of unitary man's development in constant interaction with the environment

b. Must base its practice on a body of knowledge that is validated by research

c. Is based on scientific knowledge, abstract knowledge, intellectual judgment, and compassion

d. Is a humanistic science dedicated to compassionate concern for maintaining and promoting health, preventing illness, and rehabilitating persons

e. Seeks to promote symphonic interaction between the environment and the person to strengthen the coherence and integrity of humans

f. Attempts to direct and redirect patterns of interaction between the person and his environment for the realization of maximum health potential

g. Focuses on the person's wholeness

h. Uses interventions to coordinate the human field with the rhythmicities of the environmental field

i. Is collaborative with other health care disciplines

Points to Remember

The four building blocks of Rogers's model are energy fields, universe of open systems, pattern, and four dimensionality.

The human being and the environment are irreducible wholes that contain infinite energy fields.

Rogers's Principles of Homeodynamics consist of integrality, resonancy, and helicy.

Nursing is viewed as both an art and a science.

Nursing is unique to Rogers because it focuses on the wholeness of the person.

Glossary

Energy field — fundamental unit of living and nonliving things

Four dimensionality — nonlinear domain without spatial or temporal attributes

Homeodynamics — principles developed by Rogers unique to nursing science that denote the state of constant growth and change of an object or event

Pattern — distinguishing characteristic of an energy field, perceived as a single wave

Rhythmicities — repatterning that evolves from incorporation of past changes, resulting in new patterns

Science — organized body of abstract knowledge arrived at through scientific research and logical analysis

Orem's General Theory of Nursing

Learning Objectives
After studying this section, the reader should be able to:

● Describe the three related theories that serve as the foundation of Orem's General Theory of Nursing.

● Define the major concepts of each of the three theories.

● Discuss how Orem addresses the four concepts of the nursing metaparadigm.

XII. Orem's General Theory of Nursing

A. **Introduction**
1. Dorothea E. Orem began her nursing career in the early 1930s after receiving her RN diploma from Providence Hospital School of Nursing, Washington, D.C.
2. In 1939, she received her BS in nursing, and in 1945, her MS in nursing education from Catholic University of America, Washington, D.C.
3. In 1976, she received an honorary Doctorate of Science degree from Georgetown University, Washington, D.C.
4. Orem has worked as a staff nurse, private duty nurse, nurse educator, administrator, and consultant
5. In 1958, while employed as a consultant to the Office of Education, Department of Health, Education, and Welfare, to improve practical nurse training, Orem began work on her Self-Care Theory
6. Orem first published her concept of nursing as providing for an individual's self-care in 1959 in "Guides for Developing Curricula for the Education of Practical Nurses," a government publication
   a. In 1971, she further developed her ideas of focusing on the individual in *Nursing: Concepts of Practice*
   b. In 1980 and 1985, she refined and expanded her ideas to include self-care of families, groups, and communities; the 4th edition of her book was published in 1990
7. Orem's theory consists of three related theories, collectively referred to as Orem's General Theory of Nursing

B. **Self-care Theory**
1. General information
   a. Describes and explains self-care
   b. Is based on the concepts of self-care, self-care agency, self-care requisites, and therapeutic self-care demand
   c. Promotes the goal of patient self-care
2. Self-care: comprises those activities performed independently by an individual to promote and maintain personal well-being throughout life
3. Self-care agency
   a. Is the individual's ability to perform self-care activities
   b. Consists of two agents: *self-care agent* (person who provides the self-care) and *dependent care agent* (person other than the individual who provides the care, such as a parent who cares for a child)
4. Self-care requisites
   a. Are the actions or measures used to provide self-care; also called self-care needs

    b. Consist of three categories: *universal* (requisites that are common to all individuals, such as maintaining air, water, and food intake and elimination; balancing activity, rest, solitude, and social interaction; and preventing hazards and promoting normalcy), *developmental* (specialized universal self-care requisites that result from maturation or new requisites that develop as a result of a condition or event, such as adjusting to the loss of a spouse or a change in body image), and *health deviation* (requisites that result from illness, injury, or disease or its treatment; they include such actions as seeking medical assistance, carrying out a prescribed treatment, and learning to live with the effects of illness or treatment)

5. Therapeutic self-care demand
    a. Refers to those self-care activities required to meet the self-care requisites
    b. Involves the use of actions to maintain health and well-being; each patient's therapeutic self-care demand varies throughout life
    c. Can produce a self-care deficit when it exceeds the patient's self-care agency (see *Orem's conceptual framework for nursing*)

C. Self-care Deficit Theory
1. General information
    a. Is the central focus of Orem's General Theory of Nursing
    b. Explains when nursing is needed
    c. Describes and explains how people can be helped through nursing
2. Self-care deficit
    a. Arises when the self-care agency cannot meet self-care requisites (when a patient cannot administer self-care)
    b. Necessitates nursing to meet the self-care requisites through five methods of help: acting or doing for, guiding, teaching, supporting, and providing an environment to promote the patient's ability to meet current or future demands

D. Nursing Systems Theory
1. General information
    a. Refers to the series of actions a nurse takes to meet a patient's self-care requisites
    b. Is determined by the patient's self-care requisites and self-care agency
    c. Is composed of three systems—wholly compensatory, partly compensatory, and supportive-educative—to meet the patient's self-care requisites; each system describes nursing responsibilities, roles of the nurse and patient, rationales for the nurse-patient relationship, and types of actions needed to meet the patient's self-care agency and therapeutic self-care demand

OREM'S CONCEPTUAL FRAMEWORK FOR NURSING

This illustration relates the major components of Orem's Self-Care Deficit Theory. "R" shows a relationship between components; "<" shows a current or potential deficit where nursing would be required.

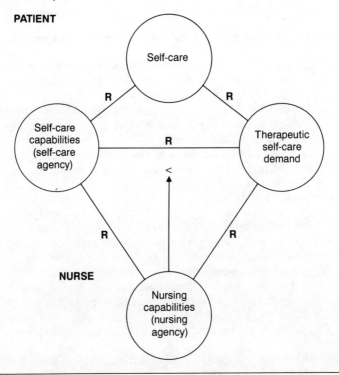

From Orem, Dorothea E. *Nursing: Concepts of Practice*, 3rd ed. New York: McGraw-Hill Book Co., 1985. Adapted with permission of the publisher.

2. Nursing systems
   a. A *wholly compensatory nursing system* is used when a patient's self-care agency is so limited that the patient depends on others for well-being (for example, an unconscious patient)
   b. A *partly compensatory nursing system* is used when a patient can meet some self-care requisites but needs a nurse to help meet others; the nurse and the patient play major roles in performing self-care (for example, a patient who can bathe but who needs assistance getting dressed)

    c. A *supportive-educative nursing system* is used when a patient can meet self-care requisites but needs assistance with decision making, behavior control, or knowledge acquisition skills (for example, a patient with controlled hypertension who seeks additional diet information from the nurse); in this system, the nurse attempts to promote the self-care agency (see *Basic nursing systems*)

E. Orem's theory and the four concepts of the nursing metaparadigm
1. Person
   a. Is defined by Orem as the patient (the recipient of nursing care)—a being who functions biologically, symbolically, and socially and who has the potential for learning and development
   b. Is an individual subject to the forces of nature, with a capacity for self-knowledge, who can engage in deliberate action, interpret experiences, and perform beneficial actions
   c. Is an individual who can learn to meet self-care requisites; if, for some reason, the person cannot learn self-care measures, others must provide the care
2. Environment
   a. Consists of *environmental factors* (not defined by Orem but interpreted by others as being outside the person), *environmental elements* (not defined by Orem), *environmental conditions* (external physical and psychosocial surroundings), and *developmental environment* (promotion of personal development through motivation to establish appropriate goals and to adjust behavior to meet these goals; includes formation of or change in attitudes and values, creativity, self-concept, and physical development)
   b. Can positively or negatively affect a person's ability to provide self-care
3. Health
   a. Is described by Orem as a state characterized by soundness or wholeness of bodily structure and function; illness is its opposite
   b. Consists of physical, psychological, interpersonal, and social aspects; according to Orem, these aspects are inseparable
   c. Includes promotion and maintenance of health, treatment of illness, and prevention of complications
4. Nursing
   a. Is viewed by Orem as a service geared toward helping the self and others
   b. Is required when therapeutic self-care demands needed to meet self-care requisites exceed a patient's self-care agency
   c. Ultimately promotes the patient as a self-care agent
   d. Has several components: nursing art, nursing prudence, nursing service, role theory, and special technologies
   e. Views *nursing art* as the theoretical base of nursing and other disciplines, such as the sciences, arts, and humanities

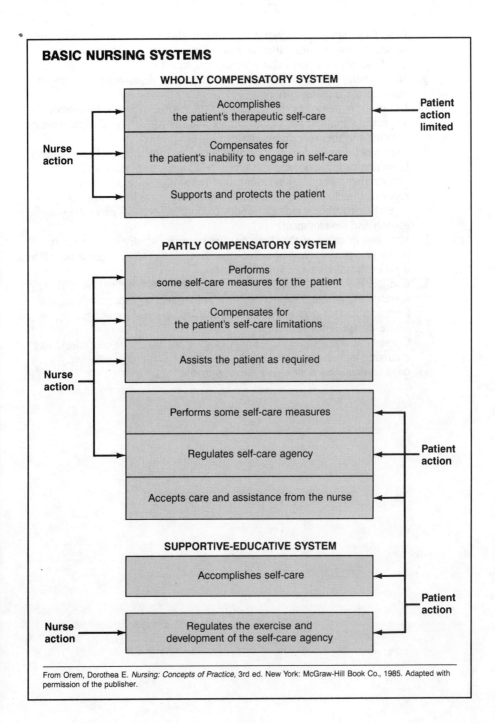

BASIC NURSING SYSTEMS

WHOLLY COMPENSATORY SYSTEM

Accomplishes the patient's therapeutic self-care	Patient action limited
Compensates for the patient's inability to engage in self-care	
Supports and protects the patient	

Nurse action

PARTLY COMPENSATORY SYSTEM

Performs some self-care measures for the patient

Compensates for the patient's self-care limitations

Assists the patient as required

Nurse action

Performs some self-care measures

Regulates self-care agency

Accepts care and assistance from the nurse

Patient action

SUPPORTIVE-EDUCATIVE SYSTEM

Accomplishes self-care

Patient action

Nurse action

Regulates the exercise and development of the self-care agency

From Orem, Dorothea E. *Nursing: Concepts of Practice,* 3rd ed. New York: McGraw-Hill Book Co., 1985. Adapted with permission of the publisher.

f. Describes *nursing prudence* as the quality that enables the nurse to seek advice in new or difficult situations, to make correct judgments, to decide to act in a particular manner, and to act

g. Sees *nursing service* as a helping service; Orem describes the ability to nurse as the nursing agency

h. Defines *role theory* as the nurse's and the patient's expected behaviors in a specific situation; roles of the nurse and the patient are complementary, working together to achieve self-care

i. Uses *special technologies,* including social and interpersonal technologies (communicating, coordinating group relations, establishing and maintaining therapeutic relations, and rendering assistance) and regulatory technologies (maintaining and promoting life processes, regulating psychophysiologic modes of functioning, and promoting growth and development)

j. Uses one or more of the three nursing systems (wholly compensatory, partly compensatory, supportive-educative) designed by a nurse based on a patient's self-care needs and abilities

k. Can use methods of helping in each nursing system (acting for or doing for another; guiding, supporting or teaching another; and providing an environment that promotes personal development in meeting present or future demands for action)

l. Consists of three steps: determining why a patient needs care; designing a nursing system and planning the delivery of care; and initiating, conditioning, and controlling nursing actions

Points to Remember

Orem's General Theory of Nursing is composed of three interrelated theories — Self-Care Theory, Self-Care Deficit Theory, and Nursing Systems Theory.

The Self-Care Theory identifies universal, developmental, and health deviation self-care requisites.

The Self-Care Deficit Theory, which specifies when nursing care is needed, provides the central focus of Orem's General Theory of Nursing.

When the therapeutic self-care demand is greater than a patient's self-care agency, a self-care deficit exists and nursing care is required.

The Nursing Systems Theory comprises three systems — wholly compensatory, partly compensatory, and supportive-educative.

The nurse uses one or more nursing systems to promote a patient's self-care.

Glossary

Illness — deviation from normal structure or function, resulting in self-care deficits

Nursing — actions that overcome or prevent self-care deficits or provide self-care for a person who cannot meet self-care demands

Nursing agency — nurse's ability to assist a patient in meeting therapeutic self-care demands

Self-care — actions, activities, or measures that a person engages in to maintain personal health and well-being

King's Goal Attainment Theory

Learning Objectives

After studying this section, the reader should be able to:

- Describe King's open systems framework.

- Identify the concepts of the Goal Attainment Theory.

- Discuss how King addresses the four concepts of the nursing metaparadigm.

XIII. King's Goal Attainment Theory

A. **Introduction**
1. Imogene King completed her basic nursing education in 1945 when she received her diploma in nursing from St. John's Hospital School of Nursing, St. Louis
2. In 1948, she received her BS in nursing education, and in 1957, her MS in nursing from St. Louis University
3. In 1961, she was awarded a doctorate in education from Teachers College, Columbia University, New York City
4. She has held positions in nursing education, administration, and practice
5. King began formulating her theory while an associate professor of nursing at Loyola University, Chicago, where she developed a master's degree program in nursing, using a conceptual framework
6. In 1971, she published *Toward a Theory for Nursing: General Concepts of Human Behavior,* in which she proposed a conceptual framework for nursing rather than a theory
7. In 1981, she refined her ideas in *A Theory for Nursing: Systems, Concepts, and Process*
   a. King proposes an open systems framework as a basis for her theory of goal attainment
   b. She links the concepts essential to understanding nursing as a major system within the health care system
   c. Her vision of the nursing process places a strong emphasis on interpersonal processes
8. King bases her theory on general systems theory, the behavioral sciences, deductive and inductive reasoning, and discussions with colleagues

B. **Open systems framework**
1. General information
   a. Is based on the assumption that humans are open systems in constant interaction with their environment
   b. Consists of three interacting systems: personal, interpersonal, and social (see *King's open systems framework,* page 80)
2. Personal system
   a. This system consists solely of the individual and includes perception, self, growth and development, body image, space, and time
   b. *Perception,* the primary feature of the personal system because it influences all other behaviors, refers to a person's representation of reality; it is universal, yet highly subjective and unique to each person
   c. *Self* refers to a person's subjective environment, which constitutes everything that makes up the person; it includes ideas, attitudes, values, and commitments
   d. *Growth and development* refers to all the changes (cellular, molecular, and behavioral) occurring in a person; these changes are usually orderly and predictable, yet subject to individual variations

KING'S OPEN SYSTEMS FRAMEWORK

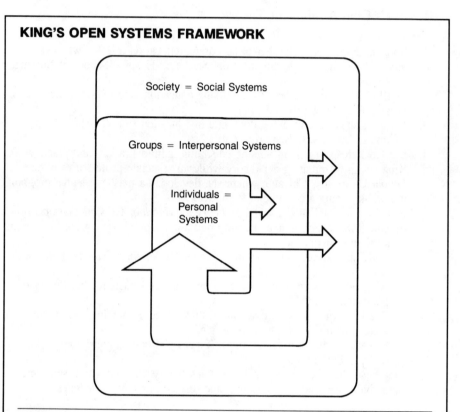

Society = Social Systems

Groups = Interpersonal Systems

Individuals = Personal Systems

From King, I.M. *Toward a Theory for Nursing.* New York: John Wiley & Sons, Inc., 1971. Adapted with permission of the publisher.

    e. *Body image* refers to the manner in which one perceives one's body and the reaction of others to it; body image is highly subjective and changes as the person changes physically or emotionally

    f. *Space* refers to the immediate physical territory occupied by a person and to the person's behaviors

    g. *Time* refers to a sequence of events and their relationship to each other

3. Interpersonal system

    a. This system occurs when humans socialize and includes interaction, communication, transaction, role, stress, and coping

    b. The greater the number of interacting individuals, the more complex the interaction; two interacting persons form a dyad, three form a triad, and four or more form a small or large group

    c. *Interaction* refers to verbal and nonverbal behavior between an individual and the environment or between two or more individuals; it involves goal-directed perception and communication

    d. *Communication* refers to the transmission of information from one person to another, either directly (as in a face-to-face meeting) or indirectly (as through a telephone call or written message); it is the information component of interaction

    e. *Transaction* refers to the interaction between a person and the environment for the purpose of goal attainment

    f. *Role* refers to the expected behaviors of a person in a specific position and to the rules that govern the position and affect interaction between two or more persons

    g. *Stress* refers to an exchange of energy, either positive or negative, between a person and the environment; objects, persons, and events can serve as stressors

    h. *Coping,* although considered important by King, is not defined by her

4. Social systems

    a. When interpersonal systems come together, they form larger systems (called social systems), which include families, religious groups, schools, workplaces, and peer groups

    b. A social system comprises the social roles, behaviors, and practices developed to maintain values and includes organization, authority, power, status, and decision making

    c. *Organization* refers to a group of people with similar interests who have prescribed roles and positions and who use resources to achieve personal and organizational goals

    d. King proposes four parameters of organization: human values, behavior patterns, needs, goals, and expectations; natural environment containing essential materials and resources; individuals who form groups and interact for goal achievement; and technology to facilitate goal attainment

    e. *Authority* refers to the observable behavior of providing guidance and order and being responsible for actions; it is active and reciprocal

    f. *Power,* which is situational, dynamic, and goal-directed, is characterized by the ability to use resources for goal achievement; power is also a means by which one or more persons can influence others

    g. *Status* refers to the position occupied by a person in a group or the position occupied by a group in relation to other groups in an organization; it is accompanied by certain duties, privileges, and obligations

    h. *Decision making* results from developing and acting on perceived choices for goal attainment

C. Goal Attainment Theory

1. General information

    a. Represents an expansion of King's original ideas to incorporate the concept of the nurse and the patient mutually communicating information, establishing goals, and taking action to attain goals (see *Schematic diagram of goal attainment theory,* page 82)

SCHEMATIC DIAGRAM OF GOAL ATTAINMENT THEORY

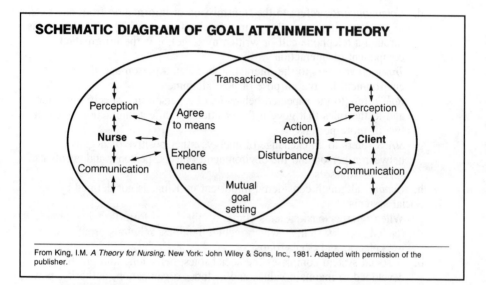

From King, I.M. *A Theory for Nursing.* New York: John Wiley & Sons, Inc., 1981. Adapted with permission of the publisher.

  b. Describes a situation in which two people, usually strangers, come together in a health care organization to help or be helped to maintain a state of health

  c. Is based on the concepts of the personal and interpersonal systems, including interaction, perception, communication, transaction, role, stress, growth and development, time, and space

2. Interaction

  a. According to King, each individual brings to an interaction a different set of values, ideas, attitudes, and perceptions to exchange

  b. Individuals come together for a purpose; each person makes a judgment, takes mental or physical action, and reacts to the other individuals and the situation

3. Perception

  a. A person imports energy from the environment and transforms, processes, and stores it

  b. The individual then exports this energy, as demonstrated by observable behaviors

4. Communication

  a. A person provides information directly or indirectly to another person

  b. The other person receives this information and processes it

5. Transaction

  a. Two individuals mutually identify goals and the means to achieve them

  b. They reach an agreement about how to attain these goals and then set about to realize them

6. Role
   a. Each person occupies a position in a social system that has specific rules and obligations
   b. Roles can be congruent (resulting in transactions) or in conflict (resulting in stress)
7. Stress
   a. When an individual interacts with the environment, an energy response occurs to objects, events, and persons
   b. The individual uses this energy response to maintain balance for growth, development, and performance
8. Growth and development
   a. Individuals are in a constant state of molecular, cellular, and behavioral change
   b. As these changes occur, transactions are made, moving the individual toward a level of maturity and self-actualization
9. Time
   a. A person experiences a sequence of events that move toward the future
   b. As the individual moves forward, changes occur
10. Space
   a. Each person has a designated physical area or territory that extends from the individual equally in all directions
   b. Specific behaviors exist for the person occupying that space

D. **King's theory and the four concepts of the nursing metaparadigm**
   1. Person
      a. Is a social, sentient, rational, perceiving, controlling, purposeful, action-oriented, time-oriented being
      b. Has a right to self-knowledge, participation in decisions that affect life and health, and acceptance or rejection of health care
      c. Has three fundamental health needs: timely and useful health information, care that prevents illness, and help when self-care demands cannot be met
   2. Environment
      a. Is not specifically defined by King, although she uses the terms *internal environment* and *external environment* in her open systems approach
      b. Could be interpreted from the general systems theory as an open system with permeable boundaries that allow the exchange of matter, energy, and information
   3. Health
      a. Is described by King as a dynamic state in the life cycle; illness is viewed as an interference in the life cycle
      b. Implies continuous adjustment to stress in the internal and external environments, using personal resources to achieve optimal daily living
   4. Nursing
      a. Refers to observable nurse-client interaction, the focus of which is to help the individual maintain health and function in an appropriate role

b. Is viewed as an interpersonal process of action, reaction, interaction, and transaction; a nurse's perceptions and those of the client influence the interaction

c. Promotes, maintains, and restores health and cares for a sick, injured, or dying client

d. Is a service profession that meets a social need

e. Entails planning, implementing, and evaluating nursing care

f. Encourages a nurse and a client to share information about their perceptions (if perceptions are accurate, then goals are attained, growth and development is enhanced, and effective nursing care results; additionally, if a nurse and a client perceive congruent role expectations and performance, transactions occur; if role conflict ensues, stress occurs)

g. Uses a goal-oriented approach in which individuals within a social system interact; the nurse brings special knowledge and skills to the nursing process, and the client brings self-knowledge and perceptions

Points to Remember

The goal of nursing is to help individuals maintain health so that they can function in their roles.

The open systems framework consists of three interacting systems: personal, interpersonal, and social.

The Goal Attainment Theory addresses interaction, perception, time, space, communication, transaction, role, stress, and growth and development.

King describes "person" as a social, sentient, rational, perceiving, controlling, purposeful, action-oriented, time-oriented being.

Glossary

Action — sequence of behaviors involving mental and physical processes

Interaction — perception and communication between a person and the environment or between two or more persons

Reaction — result of an action

Transaction — observable, purposeful behavior of humans interacting with their environment to carry out specific measures to attain a mutually desired goal

Neuman's Systems Model

Learning Objectives

After studying this section, the reader should be able to:

● Describe Neuman's Systems Model.

● Explain the lines of defense and resistance surrounding the basic core structure of a human being.

● Identify the three nursing interventions used within the Systems Model.

● Discuss how Neuman addresses the four concepts of the nursing metaparadigm.

XIV. Neuman's Systems Model

A. Introduction
1. Betty Neuman received her RN diploma in 1947 from Peoples. Hospital School of Nursing in Akron, Ohio
2. In 1957, she received her BS in nursing, and in 1966, her MS in public health consultation from the University of California, Los Angeles
3. In 1985, she received a doctorate in clinical psychology from Pacific Western University
4. Her nursing background includes work in public health, school, industry, and hospital settings
5. She was a pioneer in the community mental health movement of the 1960s
6. She began developing her model while lecturing in community health nursing at UCLA
   a. The model was a response to her graduate students' request for a course that covered various client problems rather than a few problems in depth
   b. The model is based on philosophical views, Gestalt theory, Hans Selye's stress theory, and general systems theory
7. The model was first published in 1972 in *Nursing Research* as a "Model for Teaching Total Person Approach to Patient Problems"; Neuman published refined versions in 1974 and 1980, and the Neuman Systems Model in 1989 (in her revisions, Neuman began using the term *client* rather than *patient*)

B. Systems Model
1. General information
   a. Neuman's model deals with stress and stress reduction and is primarily concerned with the effects of stress on health
   b. According to Neuman, her model affords a total person approach to client problems by providing a multidimensional view of the person as an individual
   c. Her comprehensive and dynamic model addresses the constant interaction between a client and the environment (See *Newman's systems model,* page 88 and 89)
2. Basic core structure
   a. Neuman considers the client (person) to be an open system interacting with the environment
   b. The person has a core consisting of basic structures
   c. These basic structures encompass the factors or energy resources necessary for client survival; they include factors common to all persons as well as those that are unique to each
   d. These factors also include physiologic, psychological, sociocultural, developmental, and spiritual variables
   e. Surrounding the basic core structure are concentric circles, which include the lines of resistance and the lines of defense

(Text continues on page 90.)

NEUMAN'S SYSTEMS MODEL

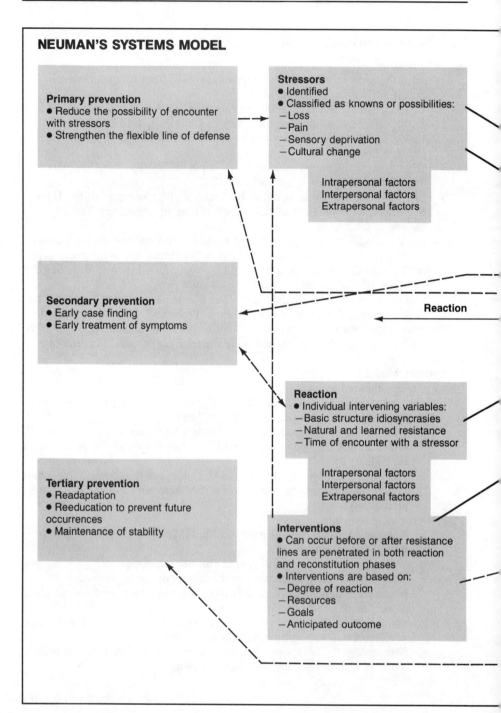

Primary prevention
● Reduce the possibility of encounter with stressors
● Strengthen the flexible line of defense

Stressors
● Identified
● Classified as knowns or possibilities:
—Loss
—Pain
—Sensory deprivation
—Cultural change

Intrapersonal factors
Interpersonal factors
Extrapersonal factors

Secondary prevention
● Early case finding
● Early treatment of symptoms

Reaction

Reaction
● Individual intervening variables:
—Basic structure idiosyncrasies
—Natural and learned resistance
—Time of encounter with a stressor

Intrapersonal factors
Interpersonal factors
Extrapersonal factors

Tertiary prevention
● Readaptation
● Reeducation to prevent future occurrences
● Maintenance of stability

Interventions
● Can occur before or after resistance lines are penetrated in both reaction and reconstitution phases
● Interventions are based on:
—Degree of reaction
—Resources
—Goals
—Anticipated outcome

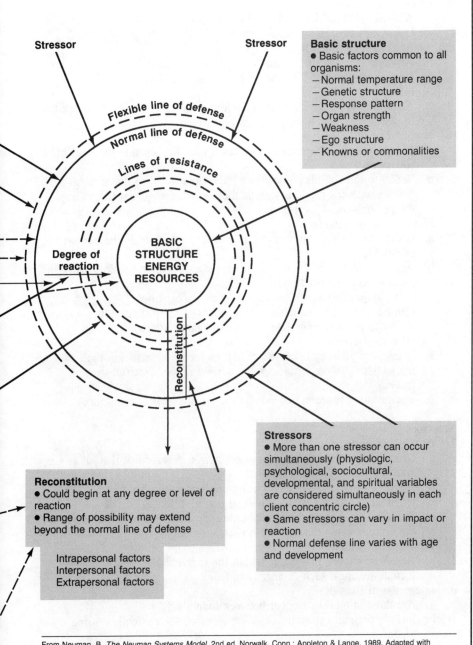

Stressor

Stressor

Basic structure
- Basic factors common to all organisms:
  - Normal temperature range
  - Genetic structure
  - Response pattern
  - Organ strength
  - Weakness
  - Ego structure
  - Knowns or commonalities

Flexible line of defense

Normal line of defense

Lines of resistance

Degree of reaction

BASIC STRUCTURE ENERGY RESOURCES

Reconstitution

Reconstitution
- Could begin at any degree or level of reaction
- Range of possibility may extend beyond the normal line of defense

Intrapersonal factors
Interpersonal factors
Extrapersonal factors

Stressors
- More than one stressor can occur simultaneously (physiologic, psychological, sociocultural, developmental, and spiritual variables are considered simultaneously in each client concentric circle)
- Same stressors can vary in impact or reaction
- Normal defense line varies with age and development

From Neuman, B. *The Neuman Systems Model*, 2nd ed. Norwalk, Conn.: Appleton & Lange, 1989. Adapted with permission of the author.

3. Lines of resistance
   a. Are the series of lines surrounding the basic core structure; because these lines vary in size and distance from the center, they are called flexible lines of resistance
   b. Represent the internal factors of a person that help defend against a stressor (for example, an increase in white blood cells to fight an infection)
   c. Attempt to stabilize the person and encourage a return to the normal line of defense
4. Normal line of defense
   a. Is represented in Neuman's model as a solid line outside the lines of resistance
   b. Refers to the equilibrium state or the adaptation state that a client has developed over time; this state is the norm for the client (for example, the person's usual level of wellness)
5. Flexible line of defense
   a. Is depicted in Neuman's model as a broken line outside the normal line of defense
   b. Acts as a protective barrier to prevent stressors from breaking through the normal line of defense
   c. Is dynamic and can change rapidly over a short time
   d. Can be affected by variables, such as loss of sleep, that reduce a client's ability to use a flexible line of defense against stressors
6. Reaction to stressors
   a. If the flexible line of defense cannot protect a person from the stressor, the stressor can break through the normal line of defense, causing a reaction
   b. The resulting reaction depends on the client's lines of resistance

C. **Stressors**
   1. General information
      a. Neuman describes a stressor as any environmental force that alters the system's stability
      b. A stressor may include any tension-producing stimulus that has the potential to affect a person's normal line of defense
      c. Stressors can occur in any number, at any time, and in different forms; the same stressor can vary in impact or reaction
   2. Intrapersonal stressors
      a. Are those stimuli that occur within the individual
      b. Include feelings, such as anger and fear
   3. Interpersonal stressors
      a. Are those stimuli that occur between individuals
      b. Include pressures related to role expectation, such as child-rearing practices
   4. Extrapersonal stressors
      a. Are those stimuli that occur outside the person

   b. Include job or financial pressures

D. Degree of reaction
   1. General information
      a. Neuman describes the degree of reaction as the amount of system instability that occurs after exposure to a stressor
      b. A person's reaction to a stressor is determined by natural and learned resistance, which is manifested by the strength of the lines of resistance and of the normal and flexible lines of defense
      c. The degree of reaction is determined by the timing, type, and strength of the stressor, as well as by the person's basic core structure, experiences, available energy resources, and perception of the stressor
      d. The interrelationship of variables (physiologic, psychological, sociocultural, developmental, and spiritual) also determines the nature and degree of a person's reaction to the stressor
      e. As part of the reaction, a person's system can adapt to the stressor; this adaptation is called *reconstitution*
      f. According to Neuman, specific interventions are used to retain or maintain system stability; these include primary, secondary, and tertiary prevention
   2. Primary prevention
      a. Refers to intervention before a reaction occurs; according to Neuman, the stressor is suspected or identified and viewed as a possible risk to the normal line of defense
      b. Seeks to interfere with the stressor's penetration into the normal line of defense
      c. Attempts to prevent the stressor from occurring, lessen the possibility that the stressor will affect the person, or strengthen the normal line of defense (for example, developing a special diet for a mother who breast-feeds her infant)
   3. Secondary prevention
      a. Refers to intervention after a reaction occurs
      b. Includes early case finding and treatment of problems
      c. Seeks to strengthen the lines of resistance to reduce the degree of reaction (for example, counseling a grieving client)
   4. Tertiary prevention
      a. Refers to intervention after active treatment of a reaction
      b. Takes place when reconstitution or some degree of stabilization has occurred
      c. Seeks to maintain adaptation and strengthen the lines of resistance to prevent future reactions (for example, initiating physical therapy for a client with a fractured leg)
      d. Focuses mainly on reeducation measures, which leads full circle to primary prevention

E. Neuman's model and the four concepts of the nursing metaparadigm
  1. Person
      a. Is viewed by Neuman as a whole, multidimensional, dynamic system
      b. Is composed of basic core structures as well as physiologic, psychological, sociocultural, developmental, and spiritual variables; these core structures and variables constantly interact with the environment
      c. Can be an individual, family, group, or community
      d. Focuses on the person's relationship and response to stress
  2. Environment
      a. Is described as those internal and external forces surrounding the person at any given time
      b. Includes intrapersonal, interpersonal, and extrapersonal stressors that can interfere with the person's normal line of defense and can affect the system's stability
  3. Health
      a. Is defined by Neuman as a state of wellness or system stability
      b. Is demonstrated by the harmony or balance of all the parts and subparts of the client system
      c. Is reflected by the level of wellness
  4. Nursing
      a. Is a unique profession that deals with all the variables affecting the person
      b. Views the person as a whole
      c. Is defined by Neuman as actions that assist persons, families, and groups to attain and maintain a maximum level of wellness
      d. Uses primary, secondary, and tertiary interventions to reduce a client's stressors
      e. Consists of three steps: nursing diagnosis, nursing goals, and nursing outcomes

Points to Remember

Neuman's Systems Model is a total person approach to nursing that provides a multi-dimensional view of the person as an individual.

The person is viewed as an open, dynamic system in constant interaction with the environment.

Surrounding the person's basic core structure are lines of resistance, a normal line of defense, and a flexible line of defense, which attempt to combat the effect of stressors.

The nurse uses specific interventions based on the degree of reaction to the stressor.

Neuman's nursing process consists of three steps — nursing diagnosis, nursing goals, and nursing outcomes.

Glossary

Basic core structure — physiologic, psychological, sociocultural, developmental, and spiritual variables that make up a client

Intervention — purposeful action used to help a client attain, retain, or maintain stability

Reconstitution — state of adaptation to stressors

Stressor — any force that may alter a system's stability

Roy's Adaptation Model

Learning Objectives

After studying this section, the reader should be able to:

- Describe Roy's Adaptation Model.

- Discuss the regulator and cognator subsystems and the modes of adaptation.

- Discuss how Roy addresses the four concepts of the nursing metaparadigm.

XV. Roy's Adaptation Model

A. **Introduction**
   1. Sister Callista Roy began her nursing career in 1963 after receiving her BS in nursing from Mount Saint Mary's College, Los Angeles
   2. In 1966, she received her MS in nursing, and in 1977, her doctorate in sociology from the University of California, Los Angeles
   3. She is a Fellow in the American Academy of Nursing, an honorary nursing society that elects nursing leaders annually
   4. In 1964, Roy began work on her model when Professor Dorothy E. Johnson, a behavioral model theorist, challenged her during a graduate seminar class to develop a conceptual model for nursing
      a. Roy based her model on Harry Helson's work in psychophysics
      b. She was also influenced by the ability of children to adapt to major changes, which she observed when she worked in pediatric nursing
   5. In 1968, Mount Saint Mary's College in Los Angeles adopted Roy's model as the framework for its undergraduate nursing curriculum
   6. In 1976, Roy published *Introduction to Nursing: An Adaptation Model*
   7. In 1984, after further clarification and refinement of the model through research and testing, she published a revised version
   8. Roy's model is characterized as a systems theory with a strong analysis of interactions
   9. The model contains five essential elements: patiency (the person receiving nursing care), goal of nursing (adapting to change), health, environment, and direction of nursing activities (facilitating adaptation)
      a. All of the elements are interrelated
      b. Systems, coping mechanisms, and adaptive modes are used to address these elements

B. **Systems**
   1. General information
      a. Are a set of organized components related to form a whole; Roy considers the recipient of care to be an open, adaptive system
      b. Are greater than the sum of their parts
      c. React to and interact with other systems in the environment
      d. React as a whole; dysfunction in one component affects the entire system
      e. Have boundaries that are flexible and open to permit interaction with other systems
      f. Employ a feedback cycle of input, throughput, and output
   2. Input
      a. In Roy's system, input is identified as stimuli, which can come from the environment or from within a person
      b. Stimuli are classified as *focal* (immediately confronting the person), *contextual* (all other stimuli that are present), or *residual* (nonspecific, such as cultural beliefs or attitudes about illness)

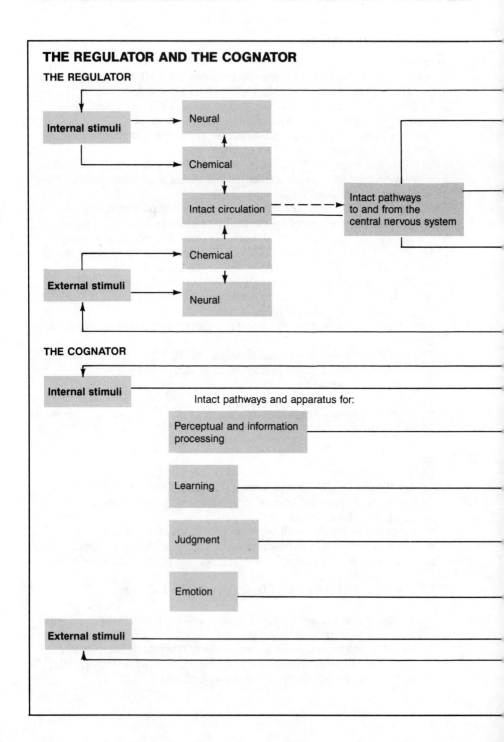

THE REGULATOR AND THE COGNATOR

THE REGULATOR

Internal stimuli

Neural

Chemical

Intact circulation

Intact pathways to and from the central nervous system

Chemical

External stimuli

Neural

THE COGNATOR

Internal stimuli

Intact pathways and apparatus for:

Perceptual and information processing

Learning

Judgment

Emotion

External stimuli

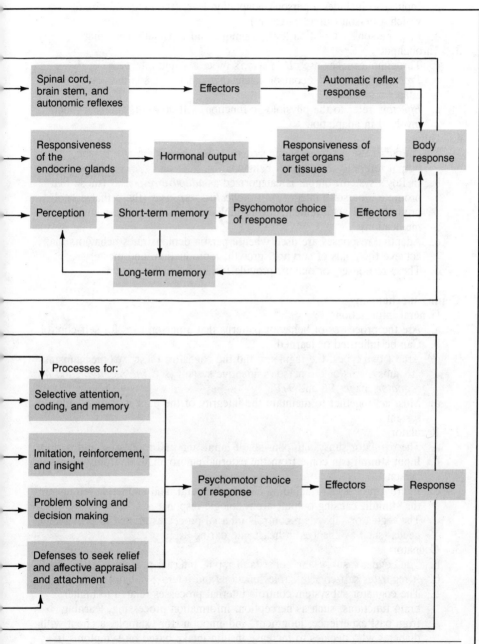

From Roy, Sr. C., and McLeod, D. "The Theory of the Person as an Adaptive System," in Roy, C., and Roberts, S.L., *Theory Construction in Nursing: An Adaptation Model.* Englewood Cliffs, N.J.: Prentice-Hall, 1981. Adapted with permission of the publisher.

    c. Input also includes a person's adaptation level (the range of stimuli to which a person can adapt easily)

    d. Each person's adaptation level is unique and constantly changing

3. Throughput

    a. Throughput makes use of a person's processes and effectors

    b. *Processes* refer to the control mechanisms that a person uses as an adaptive system

    c. *Effectors* refer to the physiologic function, self-concept, and role function involved in adaptation

4. Output

    a. Output is the outcome of the system; when the system is a person, output refers to the person's behaviors

    b. In Roy's system, output is categorized as *adaptive responses* (those that promote a person's integrity) or *ineffective responses* (those that do not promote goal achievement; for example, not taking antihypertensive medication)

    c. Adaptive responses are used when a person demonstrates behaviors that achieve the goals of survival, growth, reproduction, and mastery

    d. These responses, or output, provide feedback for the system

C. Coping mechanisms

1. General information

    a. Are the processes or behavior patterns that a person uses for self-control

    b. Can be inherited or learned

    c. Are of two types: the regulator and the cognator; these two mechanisms are subsystems of the person's adaptive system (see *The regulator and the cognator,* pages 96 and 97)

    d. Must act together to maintain the integrity of the person as an adaptive system

2. Regulator

    a. The regulator subsystem consists of input, internal processes, and output

    b. Input stimuli can come from the external environment or from within the person

    c. Internal processes — including chemical, neural, and endocrine — transmit the stimuli, causing output, a physiologic response

    d. The regulator subsystem controls internal processes related to physiologic needs (such as changes in heart rate during exercise)

3. Cognator

    a. The cognator subsystem consists of input, internal processes, and output

    b. It regulates self-concept, role function, and interdependence

    c. The cognator subsystem controls internal processes related to higher brain functions, such as perception, information processing, learning from past experience, judgment, and emotion (for example, a client with diabetes who decides to increase insulin intake based on symptoms of high blood glucose)

D. Adaptive modes
1. General information
   a. Are part of the internal processes and act as system effectors (see *The person as an adaptive system,* page 100)
   b. Are categories of behavior to adapt to stimuli
   c. Include physiologic function, self-concept, role function, and interdependence; the regulator and the cognator act within these modes
   d. Can be used to determine a person's adaptation level; this level, which is exhibited by a person's behavior, reflects the use of adaptive modes and coping mechanisms
   e. Can be used to identify adaptive or ineffective responses by observing a person's behavior in relation to the adaptive modes
2. Physiologic function
   a. Involves the body's basic needs and ways to adapt
   b. Includes a person's patterns of oxygenation, nutrition, elimination, activity, and rest; skin integrity; senses; fluids and electrolytes; and neurologic and endocrine function
   c. Is less abstract than the other three adaptive modes
3. Self-concept
   a. Refers to beliefs and feelings about oneself
   b. Comprises the *physical self* (includes sensation and body image), *personal self* (includes self-consistency and self-ideal), and *moral and ethical self* (includes self-observation and self-evaluation)
4. Role function
   a. Involves behavior based on a person's position in society
   b. Is dependent on how a person interacts with others in a given situation
   c. Can be classified as *primary* (age, sex), *secondary* (husband, wife), or *tertiary* (temporary role of a coach)
5. Interdependence
   a. Involves a person's relationship with significant others and support systems
   b. Strikes a balance between *dependent behaviors* (seeking help, attention, and affection) and *independent behaviors* (taking initiative and obtaining satisfaction from work)
   c. Meets a person's needs for love, nuturing, and affection

E. Roy's model and the four concepts of the nursing metaparadigm
1. Person
   a. Is the recipient of nursing care; Roy implies that a client has an active role in the care
   b. Is a biopsychosocial being who constantly interacts with a changing environment
   c. Is an adaptive system who uses innate and acquired coping mechanisms to deal with stressors
   d. Can be an individual, family, group, community, or society

THE PERSON AS AN ADAPTIVE SYSTEM

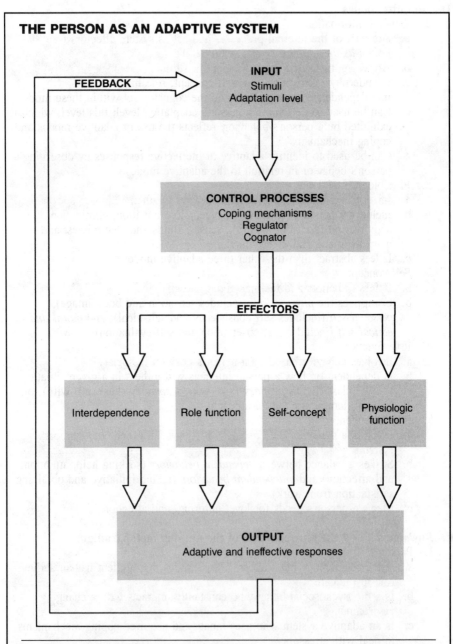

From Roy, Sr. C. *Introduction to Nursing: An Adaptation Model*, 2nd ed. Englewood Cliffs, N.J.: Prentice-Hall, Inc., 1984. Adapted with permission of the publisher.

2. Environment
   a. Is defined by Roy as all conditions, circumstances, and influences surrounding and affecting the development and behavior of persons and groups
   b. Consists of internal and external environments, which provide input in the form of stimuli
   c. Is always changing and constantly interacting with the person
3. Health
   a. Was originally described by Roy as a health-illness continuum, with one end of the continuum being death and the other end wellness; health and illness were considered an inevitable dimension of the person's life
   b. Is currently defined by Roy as a process of being and becoming an integrated and whole person; health is viewed as the goal of the person's behavior
4. Nursing
   a. Is required when a person expends more energy on coping, leaving less energy available for achieving the goals of survival, growth, reproduction, and mastery
   b. Uses the four adaptive modes to increase a person's adaptation level during health and illness
   c. Employs activities that promote adaptive, not ineffective, responses in situations of health and illness
   d. Is a practice-centered discipline geared toward persons and their responses to stimuli and adaptation to the environment
   e. Includes assessment, diagnosis, goal setting, intervention, and evaluation

Points to Remember

Roy's Adaptation Model consists of five elements—patiency, goal of nursing, health, environment, and direction of nursing activities.

Persons are viewed as open systems whose behaviors can be classified as adaptive responses or ineffective responses.

Persons use the regulator and cognator subsystems as control processes.

Persons have four adaptive modes, or categories of behavior, for coping—physiologic function, self-concept, role function, and interdependence.

Roy defines the person as a biopsychosocial being.

Glossary

Adaptation level—person's ability to respond to and cope with stimuli

Biopsychosocial being—one composed of biological, psychological, and social aspects

Coping—ways of responding to stressors

Stimulus—any agent originating from within a person or from the environment, such as information or energy, that causes a response

Stressors—environmental stimuli that require a person to adapt

Leininger's Cultural Care Theory

Learning Objectives

After studying this section, the reader should be able to:

- Define transcultural nursing.

- Discuss Leininger's Cultural Care Theory.

- Identify the four levels of the Sunrise Model.

- Discuss how Leininger addresses the four concepts of the nursing metaparadigm.

XVI. Leininger's Cultural Care Theory

A. **Introduction**
  1. Madeleine Leininger began her nursing career in 1948 after receiving a diploma in nursing from St. Anthony's School of Nursing, Denver
  2. In 1950, she received her BS in biological science from Benedictine College, Atchison, Kans., and in 1953, her MS in nursing from Catholic University, Washington, D.C.
  3. In 1965, she was awarded a PhD in anthropology from the University of Washington, Seattle
  4. She is the founder of transcultural nursing, which evolved from her clinical experience and education in the early 1960s
     a. In 1966, she offered the first course in transcultural nursing at the University of Colorado
     b. She has had a major influence on the development of similar courses at other schools
  5. She has published extensively and is a proponent of the science of human caring
  6. Leininger developed her theory from a combination of anthropology and her beliefs about nursing
     a. She first published her theory, "Transcultural Care Diversity and Universality," in 1985 in *Nursing Science Quarterly*
     b. She further explained her theory in a 1988 *Nursing Science Quarterly* article
  7. Leininger defines *theory* differently from other nursing theorists
     a. According to her, theory is a systematic and creative way to discover knowledge about something or to account for some limitedly or vaguely known phenomenon
     b. Nursing theory must take into account the cultural beliefs, caring behaviors, and values of individuals, families, and groups to provide effective, satisfying, and culturally congruent nursing care

B. **Cultural care diversity and universality**
  1. General information
     a. Leininger bases her theory on transcultural nursing, a learned branch of nursing that focuses on the comparative study and analysis of cultures as they apply to nursing and health-illness practices, beliefs, and values
     b. The goal of transcultural nursing is to provide care that is congruent with cultural values, beliefs, and practices
     c. Cultures exhibit both *diversity* (perceiving, knowing, and practicing care in different ways) and *universality* (commonalities of care)
     d. The fundamental aspects of Leininger's theory are culture, care, cultural care, world view, and folk health or well-being systems
  2. Culture
     a. Is described as a particular group's values, beliefs, norms, and life practices that are learned, shared, and handed down

    b. Guides thinking, decisions, and actions in specific ways

    c. Provides the basis for cultural values, which identify preferred ways of acting or thinking; these values are usually held for a long time and help guide decision making in the culture

3. Care

    a. Refers to assisting, supporting, or enabling behaviors that ease or improve a person's condition

    b. Is essential for a person's survival, development, and ability to deal with life's events

    c. Has different meanings in different cultures, which can be determined by examining the group's view of the world, social structure, and language

4. Cultural care

    a. Refers to the values and beliefs that assist, support, or enable another person (or group) to maintain well-being, improve personal conditions, or face death or disability

    b. Can be diverse (different meanings, patterns, values, beliefs, or symbols of care indicative of health for a specific culture, such as the role of the sick person) or universal (commonalities or similarities in meanings, patterns, values, beliefs, or symbols of care for different cultures)

    c. Is universal, but the actions, expressions, patterns, life-styles, and meanings of care may be different; knowledge of cultural diversity is essential for nursing to provide appropriate care to clients, families, and communities

5. World view

    a. Refers to the outlook of a person or group based on a view of the world or universe

    b. Consists of *social structure* (organizational factors of a particular culture, such as religion, economics, and education, and how these factors give meaning and order to the culture) and *environmental context* (an event, situation, or experience — such as social interaction, emotion, or physical element — that gives meaning to human expressions)

6. Folk health or well-being systems

    a. Refers to care or care practices that have a special meaning in the culture; these practices are used to heal or assist people in the home or community

    b. Are supplemented by professional health systems that operate in cultures

7. Modes of nursing action

    a. Leininger identifies three modes of nursing actions and decisions

    b. *Cultural care preservation* refers to those actions and decisions that help clients in a specific culture maintain or preserve health, recover from illness, or face death

    c. *Cultural care accommodation* refers to those actions and decisions that help clients in a specific culture adapt to or negotiate for a beneficial health status or face death

d. *Cultural care repatterning* refers to those actions and decisions that help clients restructure or change their life-styles for new or different patterns that are culturally meaningful, satisfying, or supportive of a healthful life

C. Sunrise Model
1. General information
   a. Leininger uses the Sunrise Model to illustrate the major components of the Cultural Care Theory
   b. The model describes how the theory's components influence the health and care of individuals in various cultures (see *Sunrise Model*)
   c. The Sunrise Model consists of four levels, the first being the most abstract and the fourth being the least abstract
   d. The first three levels provide a base of knowledge for delivering culturally congruent care
2. Level one
   a. Represents the world view and social systems
   b. Leads to the study of the nature, meaning, and attributes of care from three perspectives: *microperspective* (individuals within a culture), *middle perspective* (more complex factors in a specific culture), and *macroperspective* (phenomena across several cultures)
3. Level two
   a. Attempts to provide information about individuals, families, groups, and institutions in different health systems
   b. Provides information about specific meanings and expressions as they relate to health care
4. Level three
   a. Provides information about folk and professional systems, including nursing, that operate within a culture
   b. Allows identification of cultural care diversity and universality
5. Level four
   a. Depicts the level of nursing care actions and decisions; according to Leininger, nursing care is delivered at this level
   b. Includes cultural care preservation, accommodation, and repatterning
   c. Is the level at which culturally congruent care is developed

D. Leininger's theory and the four concepts of the nursing metaparadigm
1. Person
   a. Is referred to by Leininger as "human being"
   b. Is caring and capable of being concerned about others; although care of human beings is universal, ways of caring vary across cultures
2. Environment
   a. Is not specifically defined in Leininger's theory, but the concepts of world view, social structure, and environmental context are discussed
   b. Is closely related to the concept of culture
3. Health
   a. Is viewed as a state of well-being

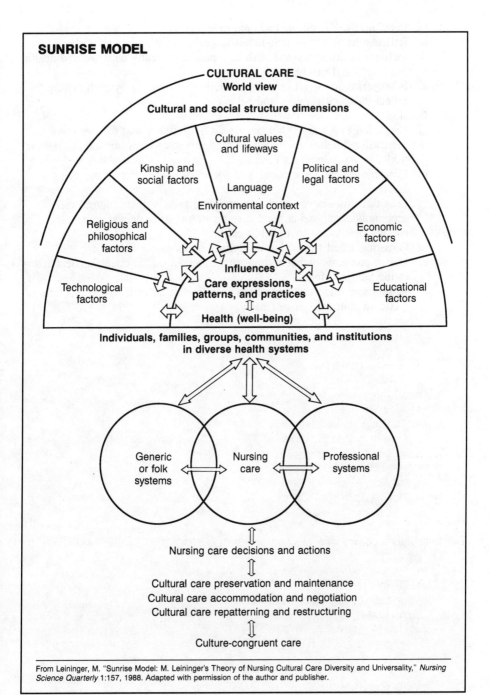

SUNRISE MODEL

CULTURAL CARE
World view
Cultural and social structure dimensions

Cultural values
and lifeways

Kinship and
social factors

Language

Political and
legal factors

Environmental context

Religious and
philosophical
factors

Economic
factors

Influences

Technological
factors

Care expressions,
patterns, and practices

Educational
factors

Health (well-being)

Individuals, families, groups, communities, and institutions
in diverse health systems

Generic
or folk
systems

Nursing
care

Professional
systems

Nursing care decisions and actions

Cultural care preservation and maintenance
Cultural care accommodation and negotiation
Cultural care repatterning and restructuring

Culture-congruent care

From Leininger, M. "Sunrise Model: M. Leininger's Theory of Nursing Cultural Care Diversity and Universality," *Nursing Science Quarterly* 1:157, 1988. Adapted with permission of the author and publisher.

    b. Is culturally defined, valued, and practiced

    c. Reflects the ability of individuals to perform their daily roles

    d. Includes health systems, health care practices, health patterns, and health promotion and maintenance

    e. Is universal across all cultures yet defined differently by each culture to reflect its specific values and beliefs

4. Nursing

    a. Is defined as a learned humanistic art and science that focuses on personalized behaviors, functions, and processes to promote and maintain health or recovery from illness

    b. Has physical, psychocultural, and social significance for those being assisted

    c. Uses three modes of action (cultural care preservation, cultural care accommodation, and cultural care repatterning) to deliver care in the manner best suited to a client's culture

    d. Is distinguished from other disciplines by its caring behavior

    e. Uses a problem-solving approach that focuses on the client, as depicted in the Sunrise Model

    f. Requires an understanding of the specific values, beliefs, and practices of a client's culture

Points to Remember

Leininger is considered the founder of transcultural nursing, which is the basis of her theory.

Cultural care can be both diverse and universal.

The three modes of nursing action are cultural care preservation, cultural care accommodation, and cultural care repatterning.

Leininger developed the Sunrise Model to depict the interrelationships of the Cultural Care Theory.

Humans are described by Leininger as caring and capable of being concerned about the needs, well-being, and survival of others.

Nursing actions must be culture-specific to be relevant for the health and care of the client.

Glossary

Cultural care diversity — differences in cultural meanings, patterns, values, or symbols of care

Cultural care universality — commonalities or similarities in cultural meanings, patterns, values, or symbols of care

Culture — a group's learned, shared, and transmitted values, beliefs, norms, and life practices that guide thinking, decisions, and actions in specific ways

Culture-congruent care — nursing decisions and actions that address and incorporate the client's folk health or well-being systems, diverse health systems, and world view of individuals, families, groups, and institutions and their effects on the client

Transcultural nursing — learned branch of nursing that focuses on comparative study and analysis of cultures as they apply to nursing and health-illness practices, beliefs, and values

Watson's Philosophy and Science of Caring Theory

Learning Objectives

After studying this section, the reader should be able to:

• Describe Watson's Philosophy and Science of Caring Theory.

• Discuss caring as defined by Watson.

• List the ten components of caring (carative factors) in Watson's theory.

• Discuss how Watson addresses the four concepts of the nursing metaparadigm.

XVII. Watson's Philosophy and Science of Caring Theory

A. **Introduction**
1. Jean Watson began her nursing career in 1964 after receiving her BS in nursing from the University of Colorado, Boulder
2. In 1966, she received an MS in psychiatric and mental health nursing from the University of Colorado, Denver, and in 1973, her doctorate in educational psychology and counseling from the University of Colorado, Boulder
3. She has held positions in private practice, consulting, research, education, and educational administration
4. Watson was motivated to develop her theory when asked to write a nursing textbook
   a. She first published her ideas in *Nursing: The Philosophy and Science of Caring* in 1979
   b. She refined her ideas in *Nursing Science and Human Care: A Theory of Nursing* in 1985
5. Watson proposes a philosophy of nursing and caring to reduce the dichotomy between theory and practice
   a. She formulated her theory from the work of other nursing theorists, including Madeleine Leininger, and relied heavily on the basic sciences and humanities
   b. She acknowledges Carl Rogers as the source of her emphasis on the interpersonal and transpersonal qualities of human behavior
   c. She also draws from the stress theories of Hans Selye and Richard Lazarus

B. **Philosophy and Science of Caring Theory**
1. General information
   a. According to Watson, caring is the most valuable attribute that nursing has to offer
   b. She developed her ideas from data on caring behaviors, discussing the similarities and differences in nurses' and clients' descriptions of care
   c. Her theory is based on assumptions about the science of caring and the presence of carative factors (structural components of the science of caring)
2. Caring assumptions
   a. Caring can be effectively demonstrated and practiced interpersonally
   b. Caring consists of carative factors that can fulfill human needs
   c. Effective caring promotes health and individual and family growth
   d. Caring responses accept a person as is and looks beyond to what that person may become
   e. A caring environment offers the development of potential while allowing a person to choose the best action at a given time

    f. Caring promotes health more than curing does; the practice of caring integrates biophysical knowledge with knowledge of human behavior to generate or promote health and to assist those who are ill; the science of caring complements the science of curing

    g. The practice of caring is central to nursing; caring denotes a nurse's responsiveness to a client's problem; the nurse and the client collaborate to help the client gain control, knowledge, and health

C. Carative factors
1. General information
    a. Watson identifies ten carative factors on which the science of caring is built
    b. These factors provide structure to her caring assumptions
    c. Each factor has a dynamic phenomenological component (developing human consciousness and self-awareness) relative to persons involved in the nursing relationship
2. Forming a humanistic-altruistic value system
    a. Occurs early in life but can be greatly influenced by nursing educators
    b. Can be accomplished by examining one's views, beliefs, and interactions with various cultures as well as personal growth experiences
    c. Provides satisfaction through giving and extending oneself
3. Instilling faith-hope
    a. Addresses the nurse's role in promoting wellness
    b. Is accomplished by helping a client adopt health-seeking behaviors, by positively using the powers of suggestion, by positively supporting the client, and by developing effective nurse-client relationships
    c. Is essential for the caring and curing processes
4. Cultivating sensitivity to oneself and to others
    a. Leads to self-actualization through self-acceptance
    b. Is important for a nurse because a nurse who can express personal feelings can better help a client do the same
5. Developing a helping-trust relationship
    a. Establishes rapport and caring
    b. Helps promote expression of positive and negative feelings
    c. Is accomplished through congruence, empathy, nonpossessive warmth, and effective communication
6. Promoting expression of positive and negative feelings
    a. Involves the sharing of feelings
    b. Includes being prepared for negative as well as positive feelings
7. Systematically using the scientific problem-solving method for decision making
    a. Is important for research, defining the discipline, and developing a scientific knowledge base for nursing
    b. Brings a scientific, problem-solving approach to nursing care

8. Promoting interpersonal teaching-learning
   a. Gives a client maximum health control because it provides information and alternatives
   b. Distinguishes caring from curing by assigning responsibility for health to the client
   c. Enables a client to provide self-care, determine personal needs, and provide for growth
9. Providing a supportive, protective, or corrective mental, physical, sociocultural, and spiritual environment
   a. Involves assessing and facilitating a client's coping abilities to support and protect mental and physical well-being
   b. Requires understanding that a person's environment includes internal and external interdependent variables
   c. Includes providing comfort, privacy, safety, and a clean, aesthetic environment
10. Assisting with gratification of human needs
   a. Addresses the needs of both the nurse and the client
   b. Requires meeting lower-order needs before attaining higher-order ones; Watson identifies a hierarchy of needs, including lower-order biophysical needs, lower-order psychophysical needs, higher-order psychosocial needs, and higher-order intrapersonal and interpersonal needs
11. Allowing for existential-phenomenological forces
   a. Permits one to understand people from the way things appear to them; their experiences shape their individual perceptions
   b. Leads to a better understanding of oneself and of others

D. **Watson's theory and the four concepts of the nursing metaparadigm**
   1. Person
      a. Is viewed as a human being to be valued, cared for, respected, nurtured, understood, and assisted
      b. Is greater than and different from the sum of the parts
      c. Must be viewed according to the client's development and the conflicts arising in this development; the individuality of each person is important
   2. Environment
      a. Is defined as society with all of its influences
      b. Provides values and determines how a person should behave and which goals he should strive toward
      c. Encompasses social, cultural, and spiritual aspects
   3. Health
      a. Approximates the World Health Organization's definition of health — a state of complete physical, mental, and social well-being, not merely the absence of disease or infirmity
      b. Is also described by Watson as encompassing a high level of overall physical, mental, and social functioning; a general adaptive maintenance level of daily functioning; and an absence of illness

c. Is viewed as a subjective state within the person's mind; each person must define a personal state of health
4. Nursing
   a. Is concerned with promoting and restoring health, preventing illness, and caring for the sick
   b. Uses the caring process to help a client achieve a high degree of self-harmony to promote self-knowledge, self-healing, or insight into the meaning of life
   c. Combines the research process with the problem-solving approach, enabling a nurse to draw from a data base and basic nursing principles to make nursing judgments and decisions
   d. Contains the same steps as the scientific research process

Points to Remember

Watson bases her theory on the science of caring and the carative factors.

The science of caring is based on seven assumptions about caring.

Ten carative factors provide structure for the Philosophy and Science of Caring Theory.

The nurse uses caring to meet a client's needs.

Watson views the nursing process as one that combines scientific research with problem solving.

Glossary

Carative factor — structural component that describes the caring process and how the client attains or maintains health or dies a peaceful death

Caring — all factors used by a nurse to deliver health care to a client

Congruence — aspect of a helping-trusting relationship that involves being genuine, authentic, and honest

Empathy — aspect of a helping-trusting relationship that involves the ability to experience, understand, and communicate understanding of another person's perceptions and feelings

Humanistic-altruistic value system — first carative factor through which an individual attains satisfaction by giving of and extending oneself

Parse's Man-Living-Health Theory

Learning Objectives
After studying this section, the reader should be able to:

● Describe Parse's Man-Living-Health Theory.

● Identify the three assumptions of the Man-Living-Health Theory.

● Discuss how Parse addresses the four concepts of the nursing metaparadigm.

XVIII. Parse's Man-Living-Health Theory
A. Introduction
1. Rosemary Rizzo Parse earned her master's and doctoral degrees from the University of Pittsburgh
2. She is the founder and president of Discovery International, Inc., an organization that promotes excellence in nursing science and provides health guidance services to individuals, families, and groups in Pittsburgh
3. She is currently Professor of Graduate Nursing and Coordinator, Center for Nursing Research, at Hunter College, New York City
4. Parse has broad experience in nursing theory, research, administration, and practice
5. She was motivated to develop her theory from her life experiences and interactions with others
   a. She drew from Martha Rogers's Unitary Human Beings Model
   b. She also used the works of existential philosophers, including Martin Heidegger, Jean-Paul Sartre, and Maurice Merleau-Ponty
6. Parse's theory defines nursing as a human science rather than one founded in the natural sciences
   a. Nursing based on the natural sciences attempts to quantify man and illness
   b. Nursing based on human science emphasizes caring and healing rather than illness
7. Parse first published her theory in 1981 in *Man-Living-Health: A Theory for Nursing*
8. She refined her ideas in 1987 by presenting two world views of nursing: the Totality Paradigm and the Simultaneity Paradigm
   a. The Totality Paradigm views man as a combination of biological, psychological, sociological, and spiritual factors
   b. The Simultaneity Paradigm views man as a unitary human being in continuous, mutual interaction with the environment
9. Parse perceives her theory and that of Rogers as representing the Simultaneity Paradigm

B. Man-Living-Health Theory
1. General information
   a. Parse developed her theory using Rogers's three Principles of Homeodynamics: integrality, resonancy, and helicy (see Section XI)
   b. She also used Rogers's concepts of energy fields, universe of open systems, pattern, and four dimensionality
   c. In the Man-Living-Health Theory, these principles and concepts are synthesized with beliefs from existential phenomenology, including intentionality, human subjectivity, coconstitution, coexistence, and situational freedom

   d. According to Parse, man-living-health and environment create a pattern for each other; man and environment are inseparable, yet each participates in creating the other
   e. Man assigns meanings to interactions that reflect his personal values; he is an open being who freely chooses
   f. Man moves beyond himself at all levels of the universe as his dreams become realities
   g. In 1981, Parse identified nine assumptions to illustrate the synthesis of Rogers's thoughts with existential phenomenology; in 1987, she reduced these nine assumptions to three: freely choosing personal meaning, cocreating rhythmical patterns of relating, and cotranscending multidimensionally
   h. Parse used the themes of meaning, rhythmicity, and cotranscendence to develop the principles of her theory
2. Meaning
   a. Man's reality is given meaning through his lived experiences
   b. Meanings change or take on different possibilities according to the lived experiences
   c. Man and environment participate in developing each other's pattern; this is called *cocreating*
   d. Man cocreates through *imaging, valuing,* and *languaging*
3. Rhythmicity
   a. Man and environment cocreate a multidimensional universe in rhythmical patterns while simultaneously living with the paradoxes of connecting-separating, enabling-limiting, and revealing-concealing (for example, a client who discusses fears about impending surgery may choose to share some feelings and hide others; by making these choices, the client learns more about the self and about others)
   b. *Connecting-separating* refers to the rhythmical pattern of relating and distancing; a person who relates to or focuses on another also simultaneously establishes a distance from another aspect of life (for example, if a mother focuses on the needs of a newborn, she may temporarily lose intimacy with her spouse)
   c. *Revealing-concealing* refers to the rhythmical pattern of relating to others and revealing one part of the self while concealing other parts
   d. *Enabling-limiting* refers to the rhythmical pattern of relating to others when an infinite number of possibilities exist; making a choice simultaneously enables (gives options to) and limits (deprives) the person
   e. By choosing freely from various options, the person relinquishes the other options (for example, a client with cancer can choose surgery, chemotherapy, or no treatment; after choosing one option, he can no longer choose another option first)
4. Cotranscendence
   a. Cotranscending refers to reaching out and beyond the limits that a person sets

    b. Man constantly changes, moves beyond his present position, and increases in diversity; this is called *transforming*

    c. As change unfolds, the familiar is seen in a different light, shifting a person's view and illuminating new possibilities

    d. Change is generated by *powering and originating,* energizing forces that create something new

C. Parse's theory and the four concepts of the nursing metaparadigm

  1. Person

    a. Is referred to as "man"

    b. Is viewed as an open being who is more than and different from the sum of the parts

    c. Can choose from options and bears the responsibility for choices

    d. Is in constant, mutual, simultaneous interaction with the environment

    e. Coparticipates with the environment in creating patterns and is recognized by these patterns; for example, reactions to the environment lead to specific values and behaviors

  2. Environment

    a. Is inseparable from, complementary to, and evolving together with man

    b. Is everything in the person and in the person's experiences

    c. Constantly interchanges energy with man as a means of working together toward increasing complexity and diversity

  3. Health

    a. Is an open process of being and becoming experienced by man; involves a synthesis of values

    b. Is a rhythmical process resulting from the interrelationship of man and environment

    c. Is viewed as a living experience

  4. Nursing

    a. Is a human science and an art that uses an abstract body of knowledge to serve people

    b. Is responsible for guiding individuals and families in choosing possibilities for changing the health process

    c. Involves innovation and creativity unencumbered by prescriptive rules

    d. Focuses on the quality of the client's life from the client's perspective; Parse describes the client, not the nurse, as the authority figure and decision maker

    e. Consists of illuminating meaning (uncovering what was and what will be), synchronizing rhythms (leading through discussion to recognize harmony), and mobilizing transcendence (dreaming of possibilities and planning to reach them)

Points to Remember

Parse based her Man-Living-Health Theory on the works of Martha Rogers and existential phenomenologists.

Parse identified two paradigms—the Totality Paradigm and the Simultaneity Paradigm.

Parse views her theory as belonging to the Simultaneity Paradigm.

The three principles of the Man-Living-Health Theory are meaning, rhythmicity, and cotranscendence.

Man and environment are viewed as inseparable and in continuous, simultaneous, and mutual interaction with each other.

Glossary

Coconstitution—meaning of a situation, derived from the situation's components

Health—open process of being and becoming experienced by man; a synthesis of his values

Imaging—making real the picture of events, ideas, and people to cocreate reality

Intentionality—man's open involvement and interaction with the world

Languaging—communication by speaking and moving that reflects a person's images and values to cocreate reality

Man—patterned, open being who is more than and different from the sum of the parts

Nursing—interactional science and art that facilitates the becoming of the participants

Valuing—living of cherished beliefs to structure meaning

Appendices and Index

Appendices

Appendix A

NURSING THEORISTS AND THE NURSING PROCESS

Because the five-step nursing process—assessment, diagnosis, planning, implementation, and evaluation—serves as the foundation for all client care, its significance to nursing theory is hardly surprising. The chart below summarizes how the major nursing theorists presented in this book have addressed the nursing process. Note that some theorists

THEORIST	ASSESSMENT	DIAGNOSIS
Nightingale	• Involves collection of data on an individual's physical, psychological, and social environments through observation • Determines the effects exerted on an individual by all aspects of the environment • Focuses on the five components of a healthful environment, as well as on the person's mind, society, and community	• Is derived from analysis of data collected and reflects the person's needs and level of reparative powers • Identifies gaps in information collected during assessment
Peplau	• Corresponds to Peplau's orientation phase • Entails a meeting of the nurse and the client, strangers who come together because of the client's felt need, such as pain or a need for information • Involves working with the client to clarify, recognize, and define data related to a felt need	• Is not specifically addressed by Peplau (nurses today derive a nursing diagnosis based on assessment data; in Peplau's time, diagnosis was the physician's responsibility) • Could involve analyzing a client's felt need to derive a nursing diagnosis
Henderson	• Is not directly referred to by Henderson but can be inferred from her description of the 14 basic needs • Involves use of basic needs as a guide for determining unmet needs and the need for assistance • Gathers data about each basic need	• Was formulated many years after the publication of Henderson's definition and therefore is not addressed by her • Could be inferred by analysis of data gathered about the 14 needs; if a person cannot meet a specific need, the nurse would identify the problem and formulate a nursing diagnosis

published their work before the nursing process became widely recognized as such; in some instances, therefore, comments attributed to theorists have been inferred from their writings. Additionally, the chart does not include the work of Rosemary Rizzo Parse (Section XVIII), whose Man-Living-Health Theory is unrelated to any traditional view of the nursing process.

PLANNING	IMPLEMENTATION	EVALUATION
• Involves preparation of nursing measures to modify the person's environment • Addresses elements that need to be controlled in the person's physical, psychological, and social environments	• Places the person in the best possible position in the environment • Involves performing measures to modify the environment, preserve the person's reparative powers, and foster the reparative process • Requires communication, including teaching and offering support	• Entails collecting statistics and data on the person's condition and environmental influences to assess the effectiveness of care • Notes improvement in or progression of the person's condition • Requires the nurse to reevaluate previous observations in light of environmental changes that affect the person • Determines whether changes in the environment improved the person's condition and facilitated the reparative process
• Corresponds to Peplau's identification phase • Involves collaboratively setting goals • Is the phase in which a client selectively responds to those who can meet felt needs • Encourages a client to feel a sense of belonging through mutual respect and communication	• Corresponds to Peplau's exploitation phase • Is initiated by a client to achieve the desired and collaboratively defined goals • Is the phase in which a client reaps benefits from the therapeutic relationship by drawing on the nurse's knowledge and experience	• Corresponds to Peplau's resolution phase • Is not specifically addressed by Peplau but is implied in determining the readiness for ending the nurse-client relationship and assessing the knowledge that both gained from that relationship
• Is a part of all effective nursing care • Should include a written nursing care plan because it forces the nurse to think about the client's needs • Involves formulating and updating a plan based on the client's needs and the physician's prescribed plan	• Involves performing activities that the client cannot perform independently or that are contained in the physician's plan • Helps a client meet the 14 basic needs • Relies on the nurse-client relationship, which allows the nurse to better understand the client's needs and carry out measures to meet those needs	• Assesses the speed or degree to which a client independently performs the activities necessary to meet basic needs • Involves observation and documentation of changes in the client's functioning • Entails comparison of the person's functioning after nursing care with that before care

(continued)

NURSING THEORISTS AND THE NURSING PROCESS *(continued)*

THEORIST	ASSESSMENT	DIAGNOSIS
Abdellah	• Involves using the 21 nursing problems as a guide for data collection • Gathers data on each identified problem	• Identifies a client's specific overt and covert problems • Is based on problems that the client exhibits • Is defined by Abdellah as determining the nature and extent of nursing problems presented by clients or families receiving care
Orlando	• Corresponds to Orlando's sharing of the nurse reaction • Is initiated by the client's behavior • Gathers information about a client's needs and feelings of helplessness, including direct data from the nurse's perceptions, thoughts, or feelings and indirect data from sources other than the client, such as health records and family members • Includes evaluation of a client's verbal and nonverbal behaviors	• Corresponds to Orlando's exploration of the nurse reaction • Identifies a client's need for help • Deals with only one need at at time
Hall	• Entails collecting data to increase the client's self-awareness and identity • Involves the therapeutic use of self to help the client become aware of behaviors, feelings, and needs related to the health status • Includes the cure circle; collecting biological data helps the client and the family better understand the medical treatment	• Can be inferred from Hall's work; the nurse would determine appropriate nursing diagnoses by interpreting assessment data; how the nurse views that role determines data interpretation • Would be worded to reflect that the power of healing is within the client and not the responsibility of the nurse or physician
Wiedenbach	• Involves the nurse's reaction to a stimulus or to the client's behavior; this reaction is based on the nurse's central purpose and philosophy • Is the phase in which the nurse experiences the sensation, perceives the stimulus, and makes an assumption about it • Includes collection of information about the realities to be encountered when the nurse acts	• Entails analyzing and synthesizing the stimulus according to the nurse's central purpose and philosophy • Reflects the client's need for help

PLANNING	IMPLEMENTATION	EVALUATION
• States the problem and goals • Is limited to nursing-centered goals rather than client-centered goals; for example, promoting safety by preventing accidents • Determines appropriate interventions after goals are established	• Uses nursing actions to meet the problems identified in the diagnosis • Involves instituting interventions specific to these problems	• Differs from the five-step nursing process because it involves nursing goals rather than client goals • Focuses on a nurse's progress or lack of progress in achieving goals and promoting the client's health
• Corresponds to Orlando's nurse action • Attempts to relieve the client's need for help immediately and improve client behavior, using automatic and deliberate actions	• Corresponds to Orlando's nurse action • Focuses on all possible effects of action on the client, according to the five-step nursing process • Focuses on the effectiveness of the action only in resolving the client's immediate need for help	• Corresponds to Orlando's nurse action; for an action to be deliberative, the nurse must evaluate its effectiveness after it is completed; failure to do so results in ineffective actions that do not meet a client's needs • Is based on observation of client behavior to determine if the client has been helped • Focuses on whether the client's need has been met
• Includes the core circle • Involves the therapeutic use of self to help develop client awareness and understanding of needs and feelings • Uses a scientific knowledge base to present a client with alternatives • Involves the client, who plays an active role in choosing from alternatives	• Includes the care circle (bathing, feeding, and providing comfort measures) and cure circle (teaching the client and family members to help them understand and follow the medical treatment plan) • Consists of helping the client to understand, accept, and express personal feelings; providing information; and supporting the client's decisions	• Involves determining if learning has taken place and if the client understands what was taught • Assesses a client for growing self-awareness through behavioral changes
• Reflects Wiedenbach's levels of realization, insight, and design • Is also reflected in the prescription component of her theory • Does not involve a specific goal, as described by Wiedenbach, although the nurse's central purpose could be considered a goal	• Reflects the nurse's actions based on knowledge, judgment, and skills • Takes into account the realities of the situation • Involves the ministration of help	• Is not specifically defined by Wiedenbach • Entails validating that the nursing help provided met the client's needs

(continued)

NURSING THEORISTS AND THE NURSING PROCESS (continued)

THEORIST	ASSESSMENT	DIAGNOSIS
Levine	• Focuses on the client; significant others are involved only to the extent that they might help or interfere with the client's well-being • Uses two methods — observation and interview — and is guided by the four conservation principles • Entails collecting data about the client's energy sources (rest, sleep, coping patterns, body system function), structural integrity (body defenses, physical health), personal integrity (ethical values, religious beliefs, economic resources), and social integrity (relationships with others, involvement in the community)	• Involves analyzing data to obtain a holistic view of the client, which is used to arrive at a nursing diagnosis; Levine suggests an alternative method of developing a diagnosis called *trophicognosis* • Is based on a client's immediate needs and problems; future problems are addressed only if they affect the client's current situation
Johnson	• Focuses on gathering information about a client's subsystems and the system as a whole • Includes data only on the ingestive, eliminative, and sexual subsystems because data cannot be collected on the other subsystems; this limited assessment leaves gaps in necessary information, such as the client's present or past health (except as it relates to the ingestive or eliminative subsystems), family interactions, education, and socioeconomic status	• Is not addressed by Johnson • Has been described by J. Grubbs, using Johnson's model; Grubbs proposed four categories of nursing diagnosis — *insufficiency* (when a subsystem is not functioning or developing to its capacity because of inadequate functional requirements), *discrepancy* (behavior that does not meet the intended goal), *incompatibility* (conflict between the goals or behaviors of two subsystems), and *dominance* (overuse of the behavior of one subsystem)
Rogers	• Focuses on gathering information about the person and the environment • Addresses the Principles of Homeodynamics: *integrality* (assessed through the interaction of the person with the environment and determination of how the two fields work together), *resonancy* (assessed by observing how the life process has occurred, its variations, and the role of the environment in those variations), and *helicy* (assessed by determining the rhythmicities of the person and the environment, the stages of the person's development, the effect	• Is the formation of a conclusion about data gathered during assessment • Reflects the Principles of Homeodynamics: *integrality* (reflected by the integration of human and environmental fields), *resonancy* (reflected by variations in life processes of the whole individual), and *helicy* (reflected by the rhythmic pattern of human and environmental fields)

PLANNING	IMPLEMENTATION	EVALUATION
• Includes setting goals that help a client attain health by maintaining personal integrity through the use of the four conservation principles • Emphasizes cooperation between the nurse and the client in planning the client's care • Requires the nurse to determine the strategies to be used and the extent to which the plan must be developed to meet the goal; planned interventions are based on knowledge, theories, laws, and concepts drawn from the sciences and humanities	• Refers to the use of interventions that help a client attain health • Uses nursing interventions that are *supportive* (maintain a client's current state of altered health and prevent further deterioration) or *therapeutic* (promote and restore health)	• Entails observing the client for areas of integrity and organismic responses to nursing interventions • Involves determining whether the nursing interventions are supportive or therapeutic, based on data collected about the organismic response; if the intervention is therapeutic, the client is adapting and progressing toward a state of health
• May be difficult using Johnson's model because of the lack of client input into the plan • Focuses on nursing actions to modify a client's behavior and bring about subsystem equilibrium	• Involves putting plans into action to achieve the goal of nursing • Entails enforcing regulatory controls to modify behavior, changing the structural requirements of a subsystem, or fulfilling a subsystem's functional requirements	• Requires the nurse to assess goal achievement • Involves checking the subsystems identified as problematic for balance and overall system stability • Determines whether planned behaviors actually occurred
• Includes setting goals • Uses the three Principles of Homeodynamics	• Is based on the nursing diagnosis identified from the assessment • Uses interventions specific to the Principles of Homeodynamics: *integrality* (focuses on both the person and the environment so that a change in one results in a simultaneous change in the other), *resonancy* (supports or modifies life process changes to move the person forward to a higher, more complex level and to prevent a return to a former level),	• Focuses on the goal of optimal health • Determines changes in integrality (integration), resonancy (modification in variations of the life process), and helicy (rhythmic repatterning)

(continued)

NURSING THEORISTS AND THE NURSING PROCESS *(continued)*

THEORIST	ASSESSMENT	DIAGNOSIS
Rogers *(continued)*	of time on and complexity of patterns, and the role of the environment in those patterns)	
Orem	• Corresponds to step one in Orem's theory • Includes examining the client's personal factors (such as age, weight, and race); medical problems and plan; universal, developmental, and health deviation self-care requisites; and self-care deficits • Encompasses gathering data about these areas and assessing the client's knowledge, skills, motivation, and orientation	• Corresponds to step one of Orem's theory • Encompasses analyzing data to discover any self-care deficits (for example, altered universal self-care requisites), which then become the basis of the nursing diagnosis • Would be worded in Orem's theory to reflect a client's inability to meet the self-care requisite related to the self-care deficit
King	• Occurs in nurse-client interaction • Involves all components of the open systems framework, such as growth and development, self, role, stress, interaction, and transaction • Gathers subjective and objective data about a client's personal, interpersonal, and social systems • Requires clear communication to validate the accuracy of the nurse's and the client's perceptions	• Is defined by King as the disturbance, problem, or concern that caused the client to seek help • Is derived from information obtained during assessment (for example, the nursing diagnosis might focus on enhancing a client's growth and development or promoting acceptance of body image, ability to deal with stress, or capacity to make appropriate decisions)
Neuman	• Corresponds to Neuman's nursing diagnosis step • Includes gathering information about a client's physiologic, psychological, sociocultural, developmental, and spiritual variables • Also includes collecting data on actual and potential stressors, basic core structure integrity, and lines of defense and resistance, as well as assessing the client's past, present, and future coping patterns	• Corresponds to Neuman's nursing diagnosis step • Identifies needs and problems (variances from wellness) by analyzing client information

PLANNING	IMPLEMENTATION	EVALUATION
	and *helicy* (aimed at accepting individual differences as an expression of evolutionary emergence and supporting or modifying rhythms and goals) • Fosters repatterning of the whole person, so that developing patterns coordinate with environmental changes	
• Corresponds to step two of Orem's theory • Involves designing and planning the appropriate nursing system • Focuses on enabling a client to become an effective self-care agent • Should encourage a client to participate actively in health-care decisions	• Corresponds to step three of Orem's theory • Entails putting the nursing system into action and assuming a caring or guiding role	• Corresponds to step three of Orem's theory • Is accomplished by the nurse and the client together • Involves collecting data to evaluate the results of care against those specified in the nursing system • Entails evaluating the outcome of nurse-client interactions; changes are made when self-care deficits persist, thereby making nursing care a circular process
• Involves setting goals that are mutually determined by the nurse and the client and making decisions to achieve these goals • Is reflected in King's concept of transaction	• Refers to specific activities designed to meet goals • Is a continuation of transaction; for example, a nurse can support behaviors that enhance a client's understanding of self or allow a client to share in decision making about care when appropriate	• Describes whether an intervention resulted in goal attainment • Determines the effectiveness of nursing care given; for example, if a client has a body image problem, the nurse evaluates the client's body image perception before and after implementation; if the difference is noticeable, the nursing care was effective
• Corresponds to part of Neuman's nursing diagnosis step and her nursing goals step • Involves developing general hypothetical interventions and negotiating with the client for prescriptive change • Focuses on devising nursing interventions to help the client attain, retain, or maintain stability	• Corresponds to Neuman's nursing outcomes step • Requires specific nursing interventions, which are classified as primary, secondary, or tertiary	• Corresponds to Neuman's nursing outcomes step • Entails determining if the prescriptive change has been achieved; if not, nursing goals are revised • Is based on client outcome, which validates the goals and acts as feedback for further system input

(continued)

NURSING THEORISTS AND THE NURSING PROCESS (continued)

THEORIST	ASSESSMENT	DIAGNOSIS
Roy	• Consists of *first-level assessment* (collecting data on output behaviors in relation to the four adaptive modes) and *second-level assessment* (analyzing client behavior to identify ineffective or adaptive responses); first-level assessment, sometimes called behavioral assessment, helps clarify the functions of the nurse and health care team • Involves collecting data about the focal, contextual, and residual stimuli affecting the client to determine the etiology of the problem	• Can be made by using one of three methods; the first is related to the failure of four adaptive modes, the second entails stating the observed behavior along with the most influencing stimuli, and the third summarizes behaviors in one or more adaptive modes that are related to the same stimuli • Can be a statement of adaptive behaviors that a nurse wants to encourage • Uses a listing developed by Roy of diagnoses related to the four adaptive modes (first method); for example, if the problem is in the physiologic mode of activity and rest, the nursing diagnosis could be inadequate physical activity, potential disuse consequences, inadequate rest, or insomnia; if the problem is in the self-concept mode, the diagnosis could be loss, anxiety, or low self-esteem
Leininger	• Corresponds to Levels 1 to 3 of the Sunrise Model • Involves gathering information and developing knowledge about the client's social structure, world view, language, and environmental context (Level 1) • Involves gathering information about whether the client is an individual, family, group, or institution (Level 2) • Involves gathering information about the client's health systems, including folk and professional systems (Level 3) • Identifies cultural care diversities and universalities	• Corresponds to Levels 1 to 3 of the Sunrise Model • Is derived by identifying a client's problems with cultural care diversity or universality
Watson	• Involves observation, identification, and problem review • Entails applying knowledge from available literature • Includes formulating and conceptualizing a framework in which to view and assess the problem	• Is not specifically addressed by Watson • Can be extrapolated from her discussion of assessment to include formulating hypotheses about the relationships, factors, and variables that influence a problem

PLANNING	IMPLEMENTATION	EVALUATION
• Involves setting goals; in Roy's model, goals are the behaviors that a client is to achieve • Entails writing goals as behaviors that resolve the adaptation problem; for example, in the role mode, a client's goal might be to make the appropriate transition to the role of spouse within 6 months • Can involve setting long-term goals to resolve a problem or short-term goals to improve the client's coping mechanisms	• Alters or manipulates the focal, contextual, and residual stimuli • Expands the repertoire and effectiveness of a client's coping mechanisms	• Involves comparing the client's output behaviors with those identified in the goals • Uses outcome to determine movement toward or away from a goal • May indicate that readjustments are necessary to promote adaptive behavior
• Corresponds to Level 4 of the Sunrise Model • Involves determining which modes of nursing action preservation, accommodation, or repatterning to use to meet the client's needs	• Corresponds to Level 4 of the Sunrise Model • Involves instituting the modes of action identified in the planning stage • Requires knowledge of the values, beliefs, norms, and practices of the client's culture	• Is not a specific component of Leininger's theory • Is implied in the Sunrise Model; Leininger advocates a systematic study of nursing care actions that benefit or promote the healing, health, or well-being of a client
• Helps determine how the variables are examined or measured • Involves a conceptual approach to designing a solution to the problem; Watson calls this the *nursing care plan* • Determines which data will be collected, how they will be collected, and from whom	• Refers to putting the plan into action • Includes collecting data and using the carative factors	• Is the method of and process for analyzing data and the effect of intervention on the data • Involves interpreting the results (the degree to which a positive outcome occurred) and determining whether the results can be generalized beyond the situation (whether the client has developed the skills necessary to resolve the same or a similar problem in the future)

Appendix B

ADDITIONAL NURSING THEORISTS AND THE NURSING METAPARADIGM

Although the theorists discussed below have not received as much acclaim as those presented in Sections II to XVIII, their proposed theories and models represent important contributions to nursing's scientific knowledge base. The following chart provides a brief overview of their work in relation to the four concepts of the nursing metaparadigm – person, environment, health, and nursing.

THEORIST	DESCRIPTION OF THEORY	NURSING METAPARADIGM
Joyce Travelbee	"Human to Human Relationship" discusses the interaction between nurse and client.	• *Person* is a unique human being who is continuously evolving and changing. • *Environment* is not specifically defined but can be inferred to include the client's condition and life experiences. • *Health* is the absence of disability or disease, or how a client perceives health. • *Nursing* is a profession that helps an individual, family, or community to prevent or cope with illness.
Josephine Paterson and Loretta Zderad	"Humanistic Nursing" is a practice theory that encourages the nurse and the client to explore and understand life.	• *Person* is a human being who is capable of action, open to options and choices, and representative of the past, present, and future. • *Environment* is a unique community of persons relating to one another. • *Health* is survival, the process of becoming all that is possible and finding meaning in life. • *Nursing* is the nurturing response of one person (a nurse) to another in need (a client) by performing actions that will increase the possibility that the client will make responsible choices.
Evelyn Adam	"Conceptual Model of Nursing" addresses the nurse's various roles in maintaining or restoring a client's independence in meeting 14 basic needs.	• *Person* is a complex whole with fundamental needs. • *Environment* is not specifically defined but is included as one of the 14 basic needs. • *Health* is not specifically defined. • *Nursing* is performed by an individual who assumes a role to complement and supplement a client's strength, knowledge, and will.

ADDITIONAL NURSING THEORISTS AND THE NURSING METAPARADIGM
(continued)

THEORIST	DESCRIPTION OF THEORY	NURSING METAPARADIGM
Patricia Benner	"Novice to Expert: Excellence and Power in Clinical Nursing Practice" presents the specific domains of nursing practice and the levels of nursing skill acquired.	• *Person* is a self-interpreting, embodied being. • *Environment* is a situation with a social definition and meaning, as evidenced by interaction, interpretation, and understanding of the persons involved. • *Health* is what the nurse can assess in the person's experience. • *Nursing* is the caring relationship involved in the study of the person's experience and the relationships among health, illness, and disease.
Joan Riehl-Sisca	"Symbolic Interactionism" addresses the interaction between people who interpret one another's actions in terms of symbols.	• *Person* refers to people who individually and collectively act on the basis of the meaning of objects that make up their world. • *Environment* is a society of interacting individuals and their values and meanings. • *Health* is not specifically defined. • *Nursing* is performed by a self-directed individual with the knowledge to act and the ability to assume various roles in a given period to help a person regain or maintain a higher level of wellness.
Joyce Fitzpatrick	"Life Perspective Model" sees human development occurring as a result of continuous interaction between the person and the environment.	• *Person* is a unified, whole, open system with a basic human rhythm, constantly exchanging energy and matter with the environment. • *Environment* is the energy field constantly interacting with the person. • *Health* is the person's continuous development. • *Nursing* is a profession that focuses on improving the person's development toward health potential.
Margaret Newman	"Model of Health" involves recognizing a person's pattern (that which makes a person an individual) in an attempt to understand the person as a whole.	• *Person* is a conscious being with a specific pattern. • *Environment* is not specifically defined but can be described as being the larger whole beyond the individual's consciousness. • *Health* is the expansion of

(continued)

ADDITIONAL NURSING THEORISTS AND THE NURSING METAPARADIGM
(continued)

THEORIST	DESCRIPTION OF THEORY	NURSING METAPARADIGM
Margaret Newman *(continued)*		consciousness, a fusion of disease and nondisease into a total pattern. • *Nursing* is the facilitator that helps an individual, family, or community to focus on its specific pattern.
Kathryn Barnard	"Parent-Child Interaction Model" views the parent and child as an interactive system influenced by each other's individual characteristics.	• *Person* is an individual with the ability to receive auditory, visual, and tactile stimuli and make meaningful associations from them. • *Environment* is all of a person's experiences. • *Health* is not specifically defined. • *Nursing* is the diagnosis and treatment of human responses to health problems.
Ramona Mercer	"Maternal Role Attainment" addresses a mother's attachment to her infant.	• *Person* is not specifically defined; Mercer refers to the mother as "self" and the mother-infant dyad as the "care self." • *Environment* is not specifically defined but includes culture, mate, family, and supportive network. • *Health* is the perception of the parent's prior and current health, health outlook, resistance-susceptibility to illness, health worry or concern, sickness orientation, and rejection of the sick role. • *Nursing* is not specifically defined; Mercer describes nurses as being responsible for promoting the health of families and children.
Helen Erickson, Evelyn Tomlin, and Mary Ann Swain	"Modeling and Role Modeling" presents stages of coping potential to mobilize self-care resources.	• *Person* is the one who receives treatment and instruction (patient) or the one who participates in self-care (client). • *Environment* is the interaction within social subsystems between oneself and others, both cultural and individual. • *Health* is a state of physical, mental, and social well-being. • *Nursing* is an interactive, interpersonal facilitation that helps individuals identify, mobilize, and develop strengths.

Appendix C

MAJOR NURSING THEORISTS: SELECTED WORKS

Florence Nightingale
Letters from Miss Florence Nightingale on Health Visiting in Rural Districts. London: King, 1911.

Notes on Nursing. Philadelphia: J.B. Lippincott Co., 1957 (originally published, 1859).

Notes on Nursing: What It Is and What It Is Not. New York: Dover, 1969.

Letters of Florence Nightingale in the History of Nursing Archive. Boston: Boston University Press, 1974.

Notes on Hospitals. New York: Gordon, 1976.

Hildegard E. Peplau
Interpersonal Relations in Nursing. New York: G.P. Putnam & Sons, 1952.

Basic Principles of Patient Counseling, 2nd ed. Philadelphia: Smith, Kline & French Laboratories, 1964.

"Theory: The Professional Dimension," in *Proceedings of the First Nursing Theory Conference (March 21-28).* Edited by Norris, C. Kansas City: University of Kansas Medical Center, Department of Nursing Education, 1969.

"Nursing Science: A Historical Perspective," in *Nursing Science: Major Paradigms, Theories, and Critiques.* Edited by Parse, R. Philadelphia: W.B. Saunders Co., 1987.

Virginia Henderson
(With Harmer, B.) *Textbook of the Principles and Practice of Nursing,* 5th ed. New York: MacMillan Publishing Co., 1955.

(With Simons, L.W.) *The Yearbook of Modern Nursing: 1956.* New York: G.P. Putnam's Sons, 1957.

The Nature of Nursing: A Definition and Its Implications for Practice, Research, and Education. New York: MacMillan Publishing Co., 1966.

ICN Basic Principles of Nursing Care. Geneva: International Council of Nursing, 1969.

Basic Principles of Nursing Care (pamphlet prepared for the International Council of Nurses). Basel, N.Y.: Karger, 1970.

(With Nite, G.) *The Principles and Practice of Nursing,* 6th ed. New York: Macmillan Publishing Co., 1978.

Faye G. Abdellah
(With others) *Patient-Centered Approaches to Nursing,* 2nd ed. New York: Macmillan Publishing Co., 1968.

(With others) *New Directions in Patient-Centered Nursing.* New York: Macmillan Publishing Co., 1973.

(With Schwartz, D.R., and Smoyak, S.A.) *Models for Health Care Delivery: Now and for the Future* (American Nurses' Association No. G 119). American Academy of Nursing, 1975.

(Co-editor, with Meltzer, L.E., and Kitchell, J.R.) *Concepts and Practices of Intensive Care for Nurse Specialists,* 2nd ed. Bowie, Md.: Charles Press, 1976.

(With Walsh, M.E., and Brown, E.L.) *Health Care in the 1980's: Who Provides? Who Plans? Who Pays?* National League for Nursing Pub. No. 52-1755, 1979.

(With Levine, E.) *Better Patient Care Through Nursing Research,* 3rd ed. New York: Macmillan Publishing Co., 1986.

(continued)

MAJOR NURSING THEORISTS: SELECTED WORKS *(continued)*

Ida Jean Orlando
The Dynamic Nurse-Patient Relationship. New York: G.P. Putnam's Sons, 1961.

"Function, Process and Principle of Professional Nursing Practice" in *Integration of Mental Health Concepts in the Human Relations Professions.* New York: Bank Street College of Education, 1962.

The Discipline and Teaching of Nursing Process. New York: G.P. Putnam's Sons, 1972.

Lydia Hall
"Nursing: What Is It?" in *Concepts of Nursing Home Administration.* Edited by Baumgarten, Jr., H. New York: Macmillan Publishing Co., 1965.

"Another View of Nursing Care and Quality" in *Continuity of Patient Care: The Role of Nursing.* Edited by Straub, M.K. Washington, D.C.: Catholic University of America Press, 1966.

Ernestine Wiedenbach
Clinical Nursing: A Helping Art. New York: Springer Publishing Co., 1964.

Family-Centered Nursing, 2nd ed. New York: G.P. Putnam's Sons, 1967.

Meeting the Realities in Clinical Teaching. New York: Springer Publishing Co., 1969.

"The Nursing Process in Maternity Nursing" in *Maternity Nursing Today.* Edited by Clausen, J.P., et al. New York: McGraw-Hill Book Co., 1973.

(With Falls, C.E.) *Communication: Key to Effective Nursing.* New York: Tiresias Press, 1978.

Myra E. Levine
"Trophicognosis: An Alternative to Nursing Diagnosis" in *ANA Regional Conference Papers* (Vol. 2: Medical-Surgical Nursing), 1966.

Introduction to Clinical Nursing, 2nd ed. Philadelphia: F.A. Davis Co., 1969.

Renewal for Nursing. Philadelphia: F.A. Davis Co., 1971.

"Adaptation and Assessment: A Rationale for Nursing Intervention" in *Theoretical Foundations for Nursing.* Edited by Hardy, M.E. New York: Irvington, 1973.

"The Four Conservation Principles: Twenty Years Later" in *Conceptual Models for Nursing Practice,* 3rd ed. Edited by Riehl-Sisca, J. East Norwalk, Conn: Appleton & Lange, 1988.

Dorothy E. Johnson
"Medical-Surgical Nursing: Cardiovascular Care in the First Person" in *ANA Clinical Sessions.* New York: Appleton-Century-Crofts, 1973.

(With King, I.M.) "State of the Art of Theory Development in Nursing" in *Theory Development: What, Why, How?* NLN publication 15-1708. New York: National League for Nursing, 1978.

"The Behavioral System Model for Nursing" in *Conceptual Models for Nursing Practice,* 2nd ed. Edited by Riehl, J.P., and Roy, C. New York: Appleton-Century-Crofts, 1980.

Martha E. Rogers
Educational Revolutions in Nursing. New York: MacMillan Publishing Co., 1961.

Reveille in Nursing. Philadelphia: F.A. Davis Co., 1964.

An Introduction to the Theoretical Basis of Nursing. Philadelphia: F.A. Davis Co., 1970.

"Beyond the Horizon" in *The Nursing Profession: A Time to Speak.* Edited by Chaska, N.L. New York: McGraw-Hill Book Co., 1983.

"Science of Unitary Human Beings: A Paradigm for Nursing" in *Family Health: A Theoretical Approach to Nursing Care.* Edited by Clements, I.W., and Roberts, F.B. New York: John Wiley & Sons, 1983.

MAJOR NURSING THEORISTS: SELECTED WORKS (continued)

Dorothea E. Orem
(Editor) *Guides for Developing Curricula for the Education of Practical Nurses.* Vocational Division #274, Trade and Industrial Education #68. Washington, D.C.: U.S. Department of Health, Education, and Welfare, 1959.

(Co-editor, with Parker, K.S.) *Nurse Education Workshop Proceedings.* Washington, D.C.: Catholic University of America, 1963.

(Editor) *Concept Formalization in Nursing: Process and Product,* 2nd ed. Boston: Little, Brown & Co., 1973.

Nursing: Concepts of Practice, 4th ed. St. Louis: Mosby-Year Book Inc., 1990.

Imogene King
Toward a Theory for Nursing: General Concepts of Human Behavior. New York: John Wiley & Sons, 1971.

A Theory for Nursing: Systems, Concepts, and Process. New York: Delmar, 1981.

"King's Theory of Nursing" in *Family Health: A Theoretical Approach to Nursing Care.* Edited by Clements, I.W., and Roberts, F.B. New York: John Wiley & Sons, 1983.

"A Theory for Nursing: King's Conceptual Model Applied in Community Health Nursing" in *Proceedings of the Eighth Annual Community Health Nursing Conference: Conceptual Models of Nursing Applications in Community Health Nursing.* Edited by Asay, M.K., and Ossler, C.C. Chapel Hill: University of North Carolina, 1984.

Curriculum and Instruction in Nursing: Concepts and Process. East Norwalk, Conn.: Appleton & Lange, 1985.

Betty Neuman
"The Betty Neuman Health Care Systems Model: A Total Person Approach to Patient Problems" in *Conceptual Models for Nursing Practice,* 2nd ed. Edited by Riehl, J.P., and Roy, C. New York: Appleton-Century-Crofts, 1980.

(With Wyatt, M.) "The Neuman Stress/Adaptation Systems Approach to Education for Nurse Administrators" in *Conceptual Models for Nursing Practice,* 2nd ed. Edited by Riehl, J.P., and Roy, C. New York: Appleton-Century-Crofts, 1980.

"Analysis and Application of Neuman's Health Care Model" in *Family Health: A Theoretical Approach to Nursing Care.* Edited by Clements, I.W., and Roberts, F.B. New York: John Wiley & Sons, 1983.

"Family Interaction Using the Betty Neuman Health Care Systems Model" in *Family Health: A Theoretical Approach to Nursing Care.* Edited by Clements, I.W., and Roberts, F.B. New York: John Wiley & Sons, 1983.

The Neuman Systems Model: Applications in Nursing Education and Practice, 2nd ed. East Norwalk, Conn.: Appleton & Lange, 1989.

Sister Callista Roy
(Co-editor, with Riehl, J.P.) *Conceptual Models for Nursing Practice,* 2nd ed. Englewood Cliffs, N.J.: Prentice-Hall, 1980.

(With Roberts, S.) *Theory Construction in Nursing: An Adaptation Model.* Englewood Cliffs, N.J.: Prentice-Hall, 1981.

Introduction to Nursing: An Adaptation Model, 2nd ed. East Norwalk, Conn.: Appleton & Lange, 1984.

(With Andrews, H.) *Essentials of the Roy Adaptation Model.* East Norwalk, Conn.: Appleton-Century-Crofts, 1986.

(With Andrews, H.) *The Roy Adaptation Model: The Definitive Statement.* East Norwalk, Conn.: Appleton & Lange, 1991.

(continued)

MAJOR NURSING THEORISTS: SELECTED WORKS *(continued)*

Madeleine Leininger

(With Hofling, C.F.) *Basic Psychiatric Concepts in Nursing.* Philadelphia: J.P. Lippincott Co., 1960.

Nursing and Anthropology: Two Worlds to Blend. New York: John Wiley & Sons, 1970.

Contemporary Issues in Mental Health Nursing. Boston: Little, Brown and Co., 1973.

Health Care Issues, vol. 1 of *Health Care Dimensions.* Philadelphia: F.A. Davis Co., 1975.

Barriers and Facilitators to Quality Health Care, vol. 2 of *Health Care Dimensions.* Philadelphia: F.A. Davis Co., 1975.

Transcultural Health Care Issues and Conditions, vol. 3 of *Health Care Dimensions.* Philadelphia: F.A. Davis Co., 1976.

(Editor) *Transcultural Nursing: Proceedings from Four Transcultural Nursing Conferences.* New York: Masson, 1979.

(Editor) *Transcultural Nursing: Teaching, Practice, and Research.* Salt Lake City: University of Utah College of Nursing, 1980.

(Editor) *Caring: An Essential Human Need: Proceedings of the Three National Caring Conferences.* Detroit: Wayne State University Press, 1981.

(Editor) *Care: Discovery and Uses in Clinical and Community Nursing.* Detroit: Wayne State University Press, 1988.

(Editor) *Care: The Essence of Nursing and Health.* Detroit: Wayne State University Press, 1988.

(Editor) *Transcultural Nursing: Concepts, Theories and Practices,* 2nd ed, New York: John Wiley & Sons, 1988.

(Editor) *Ethical and Moral Dimensions of Care.* Detroit: Wayne State University Press, 1990.

(Editor) *Cultural Care: Diversity and Universality: A Theory of Nursing.* Boston: Blackwell Publishing Co. (In progress.)

Jean Watson

Nursing: The Philosophy and Science of Caring. Niwot, Colo.: University Press of Colorado, 1985.

(Co-editor, with Ray, M.A.) *The Ethics of Care and the Ethics of Cure: Synthesis of Chronicity.* New York: National League for Nursing, 1988.

Nursing: Human Science and Health Care, 2nd ed. New York: National League for Nursing, 1988.

Nursing: Human Science and Human Care. New York: National League for Nursing, 1988.

(With Taylor, R.) *They Shall Not Hurt: Human Caring and Human Suffering.* Boulder, Colo.: University Press of Colorado, 1989.

(With Bevis, F.O.) *Toward a Caring Curriculum: A New Pedagogy for Nursing.* New York: National League for Nursing, 1989.

Rosemarie Rizzo Parse

Nursing Fundamentals. New Hyde Park, N.Y.: Medical Examination, 1974.

Man-Living-Health: A Theory of Nursing. New York: Delmar, 1981.

(With Coyne, A.B., and Smith, M.J.) *Nursing Research: Quantitative Methods.* East Norwalk, Conn.: Appleton & Lange, 1985.

Nursing Science: Major Paradigms, Theories, and Critiques. Philadelphia: W.B. Saunders Co., 1987.

Index

i refers to an illustration; t refers to a table.

Health — *continued*
  Leininger's theory and, 106, 108
  Levine's model and, 57
  Mercer's theory and, 134t
  Neuman's model and, 92
  Newman's model and, 133t
  Nightingale's theory and, 16
  Orem's theory and, 74
  Orlando's theory and, 38
  Parse's theory and, 119
  Paterson's theory and, 132t
  Peplau's model and, 23
  Riehl-Sisca's theory and, 133t
  Rogers's model and, 67
  Roy's model and, 101
  Swain's model and, 134t
  Tomlin's model and, 134t
  Travelbee's theory and, 132t
  Watson's theory and, 113-114
  Wiedenbach's theory and, 51
  Zderad's theory and, 132t
Heidegger, Martin, 117
Helicy (Rogers), 66
Helping Art of Clinical Nursing Theory
  (Wiedenbach), 11, 46-52
Henderson, Virginia, 11, 26-28, 122-123,
  135
Homeodynamics (Rogers), 66, 117
Human. *See* Person.
Hypothesis, theory development and, 10

I

Identification
  of client needs (Wiedenbach), 47i, 51
  in nurse-client relationship (Peplau), 21-
  22
Imaging (Parse), 118
Implementation (in nursing process)
  Abdellah's typology and, 125t
  Hall's model and, 125t
  Henderson's definition and, 123t
  Johnson's model and, 127t
  King's theory and, 129t
  Leininger's theory and, 131t
  Levine's model and, 127t
  Neuman's model and, 129t
  Nightingale's theory and, 123t
  Orem's theory and, 129t
  Orlando's theory and, 125t
  Peplau's model and, 123t

Implementation — *continued*
  Rogers's model and, 127t
  Roy's model and, 131t
  Watson's theory and, 131t
  Wiedenbach's theory and, 125t
Individual. *See* Person.
Ingestive subsystem (Johnson), 61
Input (Roy), 95, 98
Integrality (Rogers), 66
Integrity, conservation of (Levine), 56
Interaction (King), 80, 82
Interaction theories and models, 9
Interdependence mode (Roy), 99
Interpersonal Relations Model (Peplau), 11,
  20-23
Interpersonal systems (King), 80i, 81

JKL
James, Patricia, 10, 46
Johnson, Dorothy, 11, 60-62, 95, 126-127,
  136
King, Imogene, 11, 79-84, 128-129, 137
Languaging (Parse), 118
Leininger, Madeleine, 11, 104-108, 111,
  130-131, 138
Levine, Myra, 11, 55-57, 126-127, 136
Lines of resistance (Neuman), 88i-89i, 90

M
Man-Living-Health Theory (Parse), 117-
  119
Maslow, Abraham, 20, 27
Meaning (Parse), 118
Mercer, Ramona, 12, 134
Metaparadigm, 8, 10, 13
Meta-theories, 10
Middle-range theories, 10
Ministration of needed help (Wiedenbach),
  48i-49i, 51
Model, definition of, 8, 9, 10, 13

N
National League for Nursing
  nursing education and, 11
  nursing theory and, 12
Needs of a client
  Abdellah's typology and, 31, 32t, 33
  Henderson's definition and, 27
  King's theory and, 83
  Levine's model and, 55-56

---

i refers to an illustration; t refers to a table.